YOGA BEYOND THE POSES

Kundalini YOGA

*The Ultimate Beginner's Guide
For Kundalini Awakening & Chakra Healing*

Shreyanada Natha

Cover & design.
Mattias Långström

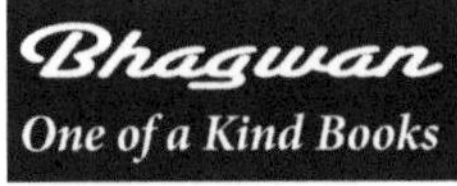

YOGA BEYOND THE POSES

Kundalini YOGA

*The Ultimate Beginner's Guide
For Kundalini Awakening & Chakra Healing*

Shreyanada Natha

ISBN 9789198839371

✳ ✳ ✳

Copyright © Mattias Långström

FREE PREMIUM Audiobook
Authentic Yoga Nidra Meditation – Swadhisthana Chakra Awakening!

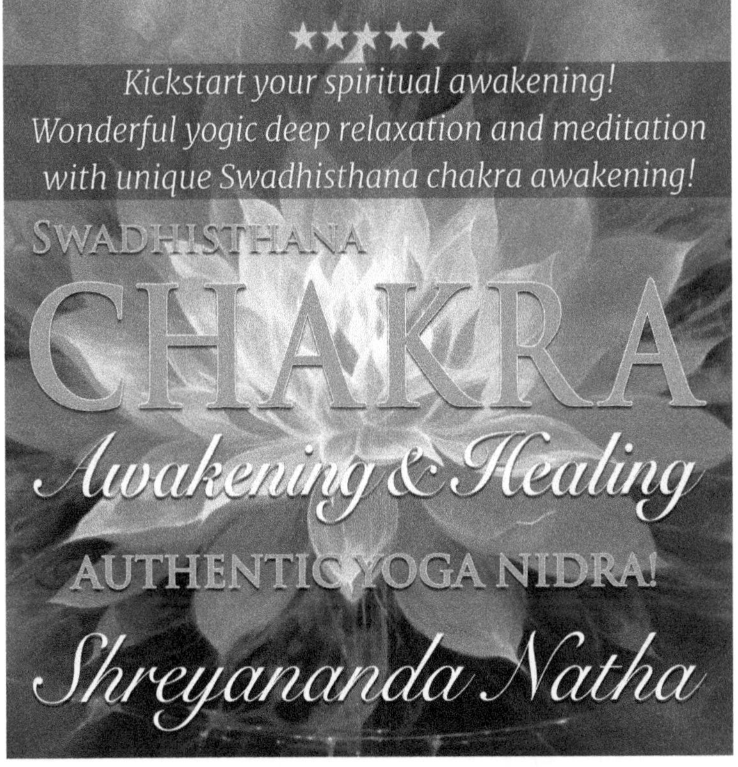

*Download the **AUDIOBOOK** at the back of the book!*

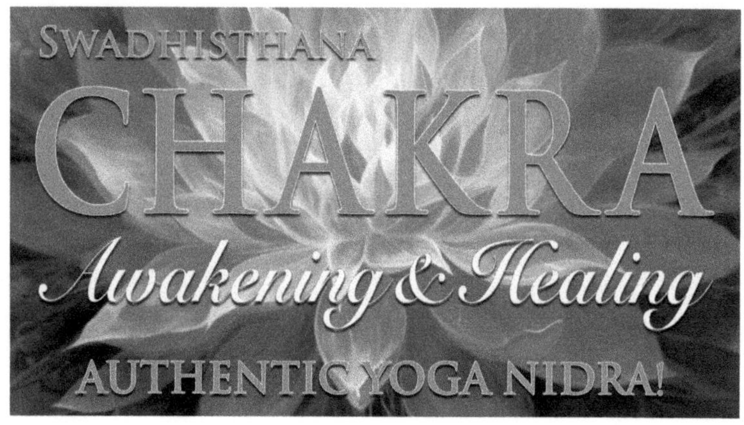

Kickstart your spiritual awakening! Wonderful yogic deep relaxation and meditation with unique Swadhisthana chakra awakening and healing.

PRESENTATION

Yoga Nidra, or yogic sleep, is a unique meditation process that's powerfully profound and healing for body, mind, and spirit.

Practitioners are led into a state of deep relaxation and the experience of our chakra system.

Yoga Nidra offers extensive benefits, yet it is one of the most straightforward yoga practices.

All you have to do is put on your most comfortable clothes, find a quiet space, lie down on your back, and play the meditation.

Yoga Beyond the Poses – Kundalini Yoga
The Ultimate Beginner's Guide For Kundalini Awakening And Chakra Healing!
Including A Premium Audiobook: Yoga Nidra Meditation – Swadhisthana Chakra Awakening And Healing!

The book describes Kundalini yoga – the knowledge of our chakras, our energy body, yoga psychology, and the process behind a Kundalini awakening. Discover all the chakras beautifully illustrated in color and how they affect us on different levels. Detect various chakra imbalances and heal yourself mentally, emotionally, and spiritually with hands-on yoga techniques for chakra activating and purification.

The book penetrates deeply but remains manageable to read, educational, and comprehensible. A must on the bookshelf for anyone interested in Kundalini yoga, the chakras, healing, Kundalini awakening, and who quickly wants to know more. The book is part of a series of seven yoga books, Yoga Beyond the Poses: The Ultimate Beginner's Guide to Yoga, that delve into the seven key areas of yoga.

INCLUDING A PREMIUM AUDIOBOOK: AUTHENTIC YOGA NIDRA MEDITATION – SWADHISTHANA CHAKRA AWAKENING & HEALING!
Kickstart your spiritual awakening! Wonderful yogic deep relaxation and meditation with unique Swadhisthana chakra awakening and healing.

Yoga Nidra, or yogic sleep, is a unique meditation process that`s powerfully profound and healing for body, mind, and spirit. Practitioners are led into a state of deep relaxation and the experience of our chakra system. Yoga Nidra offers extensive benefits, yet it is one of the most straightforward yoga practices. All you have to do is put on your most comfortable clothes, find a quiet space, lie down on your back, and play the meditation. –
Download the audiobook at the back of the book!

ABOUT THE BOOK SERIES
YOGA BEYOND THE POSES: *The Ultimate Beginner's Guide to Yoga!*

The book is part of a seven-book yoga series, Yoga Beyond the Poses: The Ultimate Beginner's Guide to Yoga, that delve into yoga's seven most important areas. They are straightforward to read, educational, and fascinating. A must on the bookshelf for anyone interested in yoga who quickly wants to know more.

MY NAME AND MY MISSION
Shreyananda Natha was the name I was given when I was initiated into the Natha Order and received the master mantra – the Shodasi mantra, after studying yoga and tantra for over twelve years, the highest mantra in yoga and tantra. It means "he who knows".

After practicing yoga and meditation continuously for over twenty years, having a yoga school for many years, and leading studies for yoga teachers, I wanted to get out more widely with yoga into our whole society, out of the small yoga room. Spread the knowledge of yoga, our chakra system, and Kundalini Shakti to anyone who will listen. What needed to be added were educational fact books on yoga that didn't just skim the surface or deal with the author's private life. So it became my Sankalpa, my magical wish, and my mission to create exciting yoga books that everyone should be able to read and enjoy. To show how we can apply and use yoga in different areas of life and achieve success and health. Here and now.

If you like my books, feel free to follow me on my social media, share and like, tell your friends about the books, and write an honest review; one or two lines don't matter. All support is precious.

Thanks!

THE AUTHOR

Shreyananda Natha is the author of popular and best-selling yoga books. He has, among other things, written one of the most comprehensive books about yoga – EVERYTHING ABOUT YOGA and the study book – TEACHING YOGA AND MEDITATION BEYOND THE POSES. He is also a certified yoga and meditation teacher according to the EYTF international guidelines. He has undergone multi-year yoga teacher training under the guidance of Swami Omananda at Satyananda Ashram and holds the highest initiation in the tantric Natha order. He frequently travels to Asia and India to learn and gain knowledge and inspiration. He has immersed himself in tantric rituals and is known for his extensive knowledge of yoga, deep relaxation, and meditation.

"There is no authority that can say what yoga is. When you surrender yourself completely and fully and experience yoga without limitations and doubts, the true encounter with yoga occurs when you become one with the true experience within you. Only then will you understand what yoga is – for you. When you are no longer limited by neatness, shyness, and artificial thought patterns that act as a filter between you and the transformation. Yoga is a cultural-historical wealth still passed on from teacher to student and helps man find his way back to his true nature. It opens us up and attracts awareness. It strengthens our self-esteem, and our person's entire spectrum of possibilities suddenly becomes visible.

Yoga is not difficult or strange. You don't have to become a vegan, a monk, or be able to stand on your head. You just need to do your yoga regularly; the rest will take care of itself. You can use yoga and meditation to feel better, both physically and mentally, but also to achieve success and develop in all areas of life – here and now."

Good luck!

Namasté

I want to thank the teachers and students I've had over the years who have made my journey with yoga so enjoyable. Thank you for all the inspiration you have given me and for making this book possible. The yoga masters who no longer live among us – live on with each new person who immerses themselves in the yoga tradition.

Sri Swami Sivananda, Sri Swami Satyananda, Sri Tirumalai Krishnamacharya, Sri Swami Vishnudevananda, Sri K. Pattabhi Jois, Osho, Swami Nirdosha, Swami Omananda, Swami Janakananda, Ole Schmidt, Turiya, Maryam Abrishami and Sanna Kuittinen.

People who all searched for answers to what they sensed through an activated Ajna chakra. In yoga, they have learned the principles behind the universe, the collective consciousness, and the creative force, Kundalini Shakti. The duality behind everything, both what we see and what we don't see. Together, we are helped to pass on the previously secret knowledge about our gunas, nadis, and chakras to all who want to become a Rishi.

Aum Shri Durgayai Namaha

Shreyananda Natha

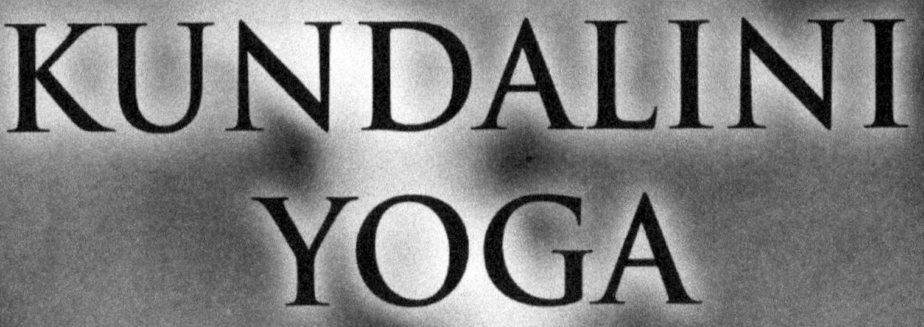

KUNDALINI YOGA

the knowledge of our chakras

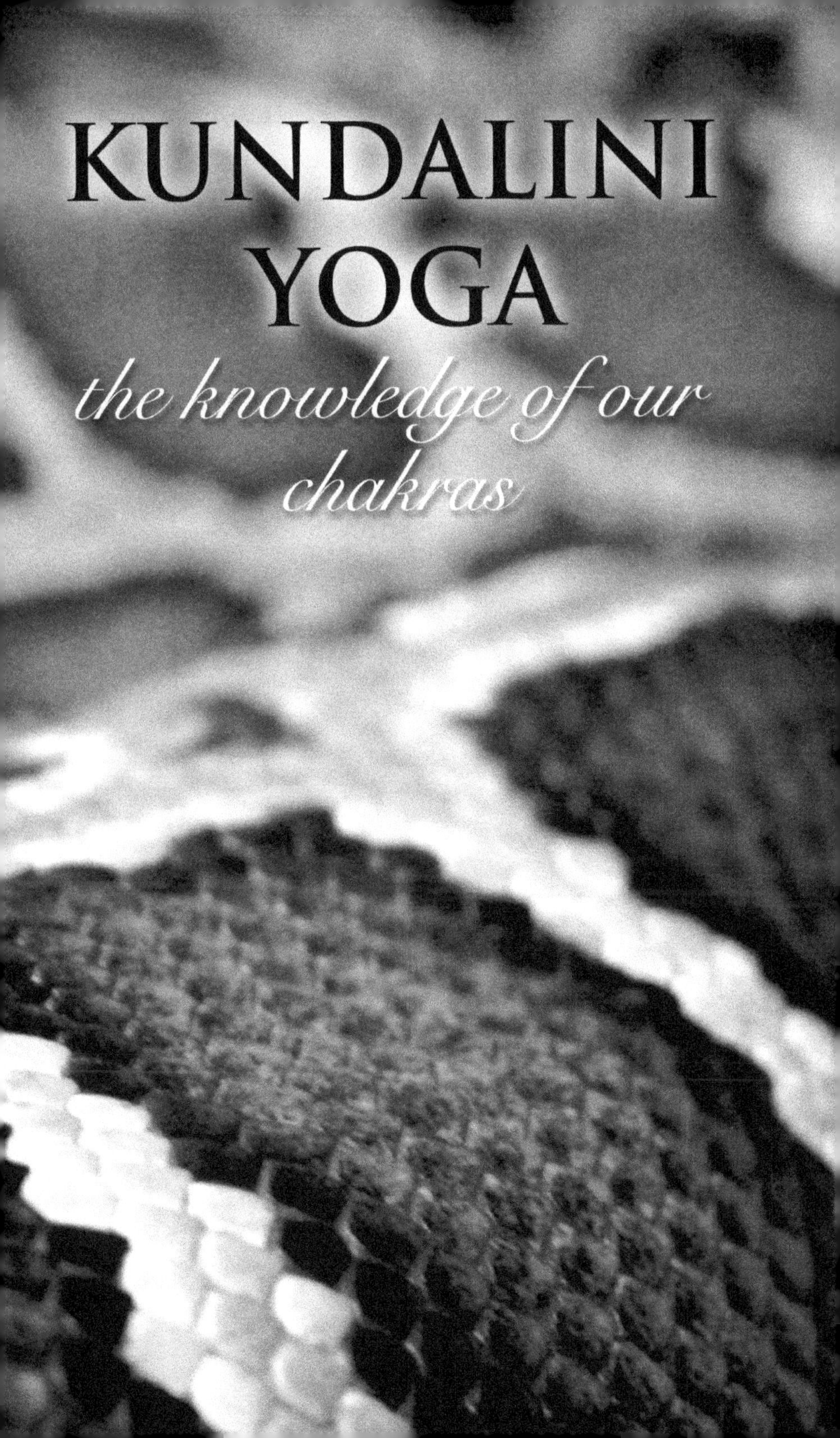

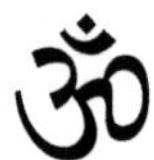

KUNDALINI YOGA

WHAT IS KUNDALINI?

Kundalini is the stagnant energy that exists in every human being. It sits at the bottom of the spine in the perineum or pelvic floor (between the urine and the excretory organs) in men and at the cervix (the base of the cervix in women). Here, you will find Mooladhara chakra.

With the help of yogic techniques such as asana, pranayama, Kriya yoga, and meditation, one can increase the flow of prana in the body and direct it down to Mooladhara chakra to awaken the Kundalini Shakti. When the Kundalini energy begins to rise upwards along the Sushumna Nadi and through the chakras, the dormant parts of the brain that are in contact with the respective chakras awaken. This process allows us to access our brain's capacity and raise consciousness.

The awakening of Kundalini should slowly be done and systematically. The body and mind should be prepared slowly. This way, you avoid any risks that a rise may entail. One should not try to control or influence the mind as such. The mind is an" extension" of the body, and therefore, it is easiest to start with the body and gradually move on with prana, nadis, and chakras.

HOW THE KUNDALINI WAS DISCOVERED

Since the beginning, man has been involved in and experienced events of a supernatural nature. When it so happened that one would feel what others were thinking and wanting, the inner visions manifested, and dreams came true. It was noticed that a particular crowd had an extraordinary ability to express their creativity through art, music, and poetry. Some people had a strong drive and zest for life, while others barely managed to get up in the morning. Man became curious as to what was the cause of these differences. In the end, through one's own experience, one could conclude that man had a unique form of energy. In some, this energy was dormant, in development in others, and fully awakened in very few. This energy was called after gods and deities. After they also discovered prana, they started calling it prana Shakti. In Tantrism, this energy is called Kundalini Shakti.

DIFFERENT NAMES

In Sanskrit, Kundalini means "spiral" or "something that is rolled up." Kundalini Shakti has thus traditionally been described as something that has just been rolled up. Nevertheless, the meaning of the whole thing has often needed to be understood. Kundalini derives from the word – kunda, which refers to" a more profound place" or a pit. The place where a dead body is burned is also called a customer. Kundalini refers to Shakti, or the power, energy in its dormant state. When it wakes up and manifests itself, it is called Devi,

Kali, Durga, Saraswati, Lakshmi, or something else, depending on the characteristics and qualities it evokes in man. In Christianity, terms such as" the path of the initiated" or" the stairs to heaven" are used. These refer to the Kundalini that rises along the sushumna nadi. The Christian cross symbolizes Kundalini rising and the resulting spiritual beauty. In all spiritual paths, whether one is talking about samadhi, nirvana, moksha, unity, kaivalya, or liberation, it is the Kundalini awakening one is referring to.

KUNDALINI, DURGA, KALI

When you can positively handle a raised Kundalini, its quality is called Durga. If Kundalini instead wakes up when you are still unprepared and not ready to take it, it is called Kali.

The goddess Kali is illustrated as naked black and wears a rosary of one hundred and eight human skulls representing memories from previous lives. Her blood-red outstretched tongue symbolizes raja guna, whose circular movement pattern powers all creative activity. She wants to urge Sadhakas to take control of raja guna.

Durga is a beautiful goddess who is illustrated riding a tiger. She has eight arms that represent the eightfold elements. She wears a rosary with fifty-two human skulls that symbolize her wisdom, power, and the fifty-two letters of the Sanskrit alphabet. Durga eliminates all the evil consequences that life can carry and comes with strength and peace. This force is released from Mooladhara chakra.

KUNDALINI PHYSIOLOGY

When Kundalini begins to rise, it passes different phases on its way up to the cosmic consciousness – Shiva, where they finally merge. The highest consciousness – Shiva, has its seat in Sahasrara chakra – the super consciousness, at the top of the head. This seat is called Hiranyagarbha – the womb of consciousness in the Vedic texts and Tantrism. It is connected to the pituitary gland. Just below is another psychic center called the Ajna chakra, connected to the pineal gland, the seat of intuitive consciousness. It is located at the top of the spine and the height of the eyebrow center – bhrumadhya. Ajna chakra is essential as it is connected to the Mooladhara and Sahasrara chakra.

Chakras are energy vortices that are experienced to vibrate and rotate at different speeds. There are thousands of chakras in the human body. In tantra and yoga, only a few are used for filling the entire spectrum of human evolution and life – physically and mentally, from the rough to the polished. Six chakras have a direct connection to the dormant parts of the brain.

Through nadis, energy flows to and from the chakras. Nadis are channels where prana (vital) and mana (mental) ener-

gy flows through and out to all parts of the body. There are about seventy-two thousand nadis. Three of these are extra important as they control the flow of prana and the consciousness of all other nadis. These are ida, pingala, and sushumna. Ida controls all the mental activity, and pingala controls all the vital activity. Ida is known as the moon, and pingala as the sun. Sushumna is the channel for the flow of spiritual consciousness. Ida and pingala do not flow in the body simultaneously but alternate. When the left nostril is open, ida nadi flows; when the right nostril is available, the pingala flows. When the pingala flows, the left part of the brain is active, and when the ida flows, the right part is active. In this way, nadis control our brain, way of acting, and consciousness.

Suppose you can get prana and chitta, ie. ida and pingala flow simultaneously; you can get both halves of the brain to cooperate in thinking and action. This does not happen in our everyday daily lives. For this to happen, it is required that the sushumna is in contact with Kundalini Shakti.

Sushumna nadi is like a hollow tube with three more tubes in it. One is more subtle than the other. These tubes, or nadis, are called sushumna (denotes tamas), vajrini (denotes rajas), chitrini (denotes sattva) and Brahma (represents consciousness). The highest consciousness born of Kundalini Shakti passes through Brahma.

When Kundalini wakes up, the sushumna passes up to the Ajna chakra. Mooladhara chakra acts as a powerful engine. To start this engine, pranic energy is needed, and it is created with the help of pranayamas. The prana is then directed downwards in the body to the Mooladhara chakra. From there, it is then directed upwards towards the Ajna chakra. If the sushumna nadi is not open, the energy cannot be distributed, which means that the prana remains in the Mooladhara chakra.

Ida and pingala nadi are constantly flowing, but their power is weak. It is only when the sushumna is awakened that enlightenment can take place. Kundalini yoga is based on reviving the sushumna; when awakened, contact between the highest and lowest levels of consciousness is enabled. Then Kundalini can wake up and rise from Mooladhara up along the Sushumna and become one with Shiva in Sahasrara.

THE MYSTICAL TREE

In the Bhagavad Gita, you can read about the immortal tree that grows up and down, with the roots up and the leaves and branches down. It is said that he who knows the tree also knows the truth of life. This tree is found in the human body and nervous system. The tree leaves symbolize thoughts, feelings, obstacles, etc.. The roots and the spine of the trunk represent the brain. You have to climb from the top of the tree (in this case, from the root) and up to the roots. In

Kabbalah, this tree is called the" tree of life." In the Bible, it is called the" Tree of Knowledge." Anyone who tries to move upwards from Mooladhara chakra to Sahasrara chakra thus climbs to the roots.

KUNDALINI AND OUR BRAIN

Humans often use only a tenth of the brain's total capacity. This small part stores our knowledge of what we think and do. The rest is known as the dormant and inactive part of the brain. It is passive because the energy is not enough to keep it awake. The active part of the brain gets its power from ida and pingala nadi, while the dormant portion only has access to pingala, i.e., prana, or life energy. It lacks conscious energy, i.e., ida or manas.

To awaken the sleeping part of the brain, we must charge the front part of the brain with prana and consciousness. We must also awaken sushumna nadi. We do this by practicing pranayamas regularly for an extended period. With the help of Kundalini yoga, one could discover that the different parts of the brain are connected to our chakras. To access dormant parts of the brain, one must work on awakening the chakras in the body. Chakras can be described as switches.

In the same way, the Mooladhara chakra is used as a" switch" to awaken Kundalini, which has its seat in Sahasrara, but most of us find it easier to get in touch with Moolad-

hara chakra. Each chakra works individually. This means that if Kundalini wakes up in Mooladhara, it goes straight up to Sahasrara. Or, if it wakes up in Swadhisthana, it also goes from there straight up to Sahasrara. Kundalini can be awakened in a chakra or collectively in all chakras simultaneously. When Kundalini awakens in an individual chakra, the consciousness is filled with what is characteristic of that particular chakra.

WHAT KUNDALINI SHAKTI IS

There are many different descriptions of what Kundalini Shakti is. Many yogis believe that Kundalini Shakti is pranic energy that flows through the Sushumna associated with the spine. They believe that Kundalini is part of the pranic flow in our energy body and that there is no physical/anatomical equivalent.

Other yogis experience Kundalini as part of the signals that flow along the nerve pathways and travel along the spinal cord up to specific brain parts. However, most agree that Kundalini's psychophysiological experience manifests in the spine.

METHODS FOR AWAKENING:

In Tantrism, various techniques are used to awaken Kundalini Shakti. These can be practiced individually or in combination with each other.

AWAKENED IN CONNECTION WITH BIRTH

A few children are born with an already awake Kundalini. These children look at life very clearly and have a highly developed way of thinking and a very unusual way of looking at life. They often have no normal social relationship with their parents because they see them as" those who gave them life."

MANTRA

It is a powerful, gentle, and risk-free method. However, it requires patience, time, discipline, and regularity. Through mantra repetition and the vibration of sound, a wave of patterns is created that affects the mind. The physical, mental, and emotional body is cleansed. It is essential to focus the mantra on something by, for example, focusing on the tip of the nose or a chakra.

TAPASYA

It is a psychological procedure where you start a process that, from the root, eliminates terrible habits that have created weakness and hindered development and willpower. Willpower is the core of tapasya. To enable growth and willpower, you want to curb the inner fire, live in celibacy, say no to lust, be restrained, and deny your desires.

ASUHADHI – Using Herbs

This is the fastest and most effective method besides tantric initiation. It should not be confused with the use of drugs. Asuhadhi is a risky method that should only be done under the guidance of a guru.

PSYCHEDELIA – with the help of psychoactive drugs.

Ayahuasca, LSD, DMT, magic mushrooms, etc., are all psychoactive drugs used to expand the mind and to awaken Kundalini Shakti quickly. Shamans have been using mind-expanding drugs since ancient times. There are significant risks associated with developing the mind using drugs. Psychoses, delusions, and other unpleasant mental experiences can be triggered, even if they do not create a physical dependence. Awakening Kundalini Shakti too quickly and powerfully without being prepared is possible. Be cautious. Take it slow.

RAJA YOGA

With Raja yoga, one merges the individual consciousness with the universal superconscious. This is done step by step with the help of concentration, meditation, and the experience of unity with the absolute and highest self. When you focus and calm your mind, the sushumna opens, enabling Kundalini's rising. This mild method is experienced as problematic by many because it requires a lot of patience and discipline.

PRANAYAMA

Pranayamas are very powerful. Kundalini can be awakened very quickly if you are well prepared, live healthy, and have a calm and safe place to practice breathing exercises. Pranayamas strongly affect the body, creating heat while lowering the temperature in the inner body. Breathing changes the pattern of brain waves. It is essential to cleanse the body with the help of shatkarmas before entering the process to handle the rapid changes better. Breathing is the link between Hatha and Kundalini yoga.

KRIYA YOGA

This is the simplest method for people living in the modern world. Here, you do not have to confront the mind like, e.g., Raja yoga. People who are Sattvic may find it easy to awaken Kundalini through Raja yoga. Still, if you have a tumultuous mind that is constantly in motion, it only creates even more tension, guilt, complexity, and sometimes even schizophrenia. When practicing Kriya yoga, Kundalini Shakti is awakened slowly and methodically.

TANTRIC INITIATION

This method requires an understanding of what Shiva and Shakti stand for. You have to change your approach to passions and desires in life. Under the guidance of a guru, this is the fastest way to Kundalini awakening.

SHAKTIPAT

A guru performs this method. One experiences a temporary state of awakening – samadhi.

SURRENDER YOURSELF

This path means that one does not strive to awaken Kundalini Shakti. You let it happen when it happens and if it happens. It is believed that a strong enough will can arouse Kundalini.

PREPARATIONS

It is essential to learn Kundalini yoga from a competent teacher so that one knows for sure that the process is going the right way. It is also necessary to be physically, mentally, and emotionally prepared. Waking up Kundalini Shakti can take time; you can count on it being a long process. However, nothing says that Kundalini cannot wake up quickly. What takes time is learning to keep the Kundalini alive.

The Sushumna must be open; otherwise, Kundalini will rise along the ida or pingala, leading to complications. The elements, chakras, and nadis must also be purified for Kundalini to flow freely. This is done with the help of asanas, pranayamas and Hatha yoga shatkarmas.

Surya namaskar and surya bheda pranayama cleanses pingala nadi. Shatkarmas and pranayamas open up the sus-

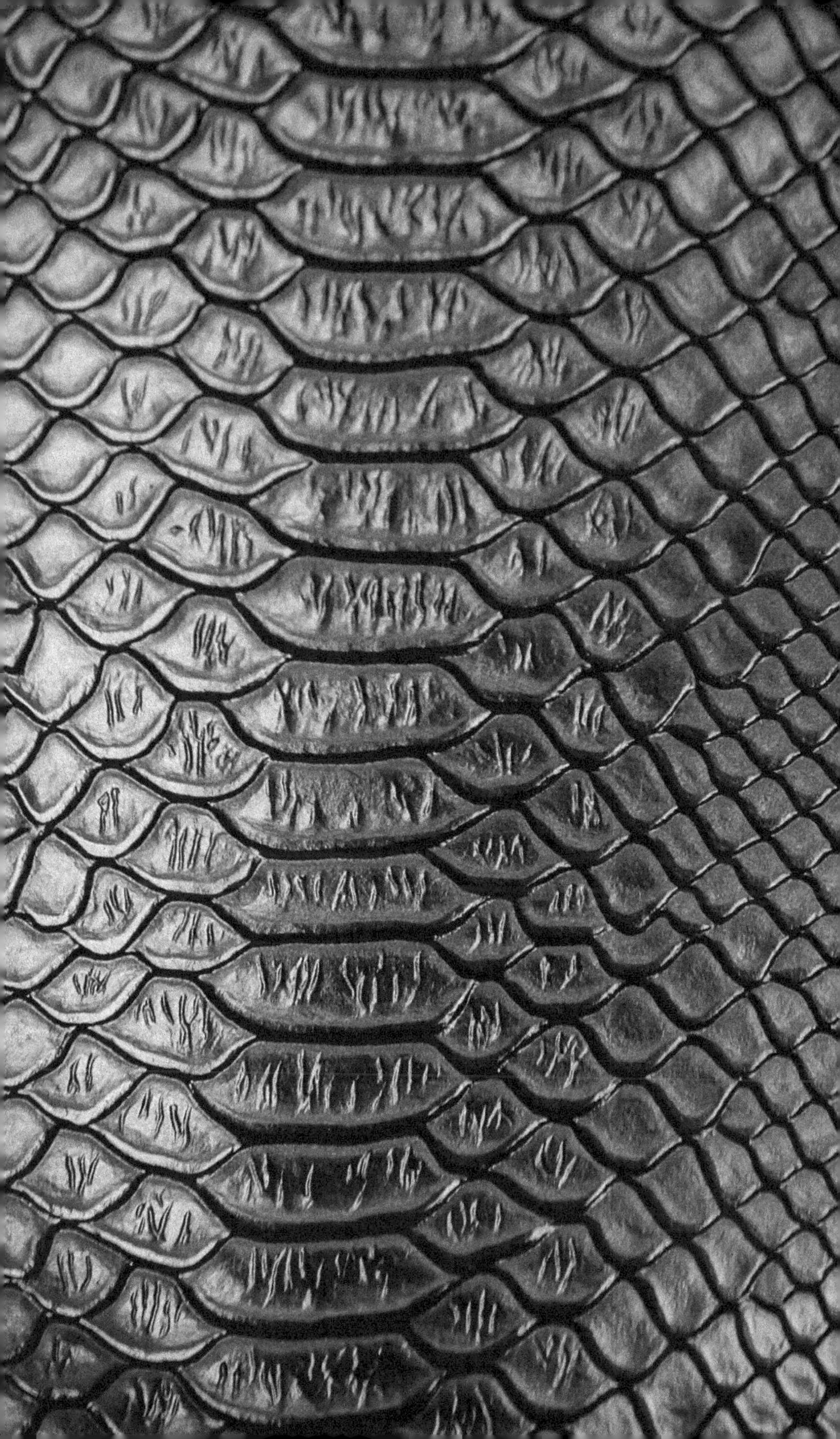

humna. You start by cleaning the elements with shatkarmas. Then continue with asanas and pranayamas. After that, you can continue with mudras and bandhas. Then, you are ready to start with Kriya yoga.

KARMA YOGA

Karma yoga is an essential part of spiritual development. Without Karma yoga, evolution will stop no matter what method one follows. Karma yoga prepares the mind. Positive and negative partners become visible, consciousness is broadened, and concentration is strengthened. Karma yoga is not a direct cause of Kundalini awakening but an essential part of the process.

DIFFERENT AWAKENINGS

It is crucial to distinguish between the awakening of Kundalini, chakras, and sushumna nadi. It should also be possible to differentiate between an awakening between Mooladhara and Kundalini. The first step in awakening Kundalini Shakti is to create harmony between ida and pingala nadi. The next step is to awaken the chakra system, which leads to the sushumna opening and allows the Kundalini Shakti to wake up.

You do not have to worry about negative consequences when the process occurs in this order. If Kundalini instead wakes up before the sushumna is open, the energy will remain in the Mooladhara chakra and create sexual and neurotic dis-

orders. Should any chakra not be available, Kundalini will get stuck in its path and create stagnation in development.

Harmony between ida and pingala nadi:

Pingala stands for vital energy in the body. Ida stands for conscious energy. These two nadis control the brain's two hemispheres, which in turn control all activity in the body. It is not the awakening of these two that one strives for but the synchronization between them. As is well known, these control the body's temperature, digestion, hormonal secretion, brain waves, and the whole body's system. Lousy food and lifestyle disturbs and creates an imbalance between them, which leads to physical and mental illness. Sushumna can only wake up when ida and pingala flow in harmony. Hatha, pranayamas, and Raja yoga are the best methods to balance ida and pingala—especially nadi shodhana.

Awaken the chakras:

All chakras must be balanced before the sushumna can wake up. Every little part of the body is connected to a chakra. Asanas open up the chakras in a gentle way. Sometimes, a chakra can open quickly. Then feelings of fear, anxiety, passion, depression, etc., can emerge that have connections to previous experiences from previous lives.

Awaken the sushumna:

It takes a lot of patience to awaken the sushumna nadi. You can expect to have experiences of a more intense nature than those that come when a chakra is awakened. These experiences are often entirely illogical and strange. Hatha yoga and pranayamas are essential for awakening sushumna nadi.

KUNDALINI SINKS IN

After a rise, Kundalini will fall again. But the mind and consciousness will still be affected and changed. You get a higher state of consciousness. Our whole lives and thoughts are concerned—emotions, body, and mind. Kundalini will be what characterizes life.

When Shiva and Shakti become one in Sahasrara chakra, one experiences samadhi, and silent parts of the brain wake up. In this state, one is entirely unaware of opposites, man and woman, Shiva and Shakti – everything is the same. During the experience of samadhi, Bindu develops. Bindu means point and encompasses the entire cosmos. It is the seat of human intelligence and all creation. After a while, the Bindu is divided into two, and the duality of Shiva and Shakti becomes a reality again.

Samadhi can be likened to the condition of an infant. One does not know the difference between a man and a woman, and there is no physical or sexual difference. They separate when Shiva and Shakti return to the rough plane, down to the Mooladhara chakra. Duality exists in the mind in the world that consists of name and form but not in samadhi.

When Kundalini sinks, and you return to physical reality, you do it with a changed consciousness. You may live with the same patterns, desires, and passions. What makes the difference is that you observe life as if it were a spectacle.

You are in the theater of life as before but as a spectator. The changed consciousness is manifested through one. You are in contact with the parts of the brain that were previously silent. One is in contact with the universe's knowledge, power, and wisdom.

THE EXPERIENCE OF THE AWAKENING

A Kundalini rise can be likened to an explosion that takes you from one plane of consciousness to another plane of being. You travel through the borderland where perceptions, feelings, and experiences change character. It is a journey between what you have experienced and the inexperienced.

The awakening takes place step by step and can take time. The preliminary awakening, usually the first step, is the experience of light at bhrumadhya. This usually develops over a long period in a very mild way and rarely creates any negative experiences. After a while, your appetite and need for sleep may decrease, and your mind is still. When the Kundalini rise finally takes place, it happens with power, and sometimes, you can experience things that are difficult to comprehend. One of the most common experiences is feeling" a current" along the spine. One can experience a burning sensation in Mooladhara and an energy flowing up and down along the Sushumna. You can also hear sounds in the form of drums, bells, music, birds, and flutes. You can also experience anger, passion, and other repressed emotions that emerge. This usually passes within a few days. Some develop siddhis, which after a while also disappear.

You can lose your appetite for weeks, become depressed, lose interest in life, and experience everything as very sad at the same time as the mind can become very mobile and creative. You might start writing poetry, creating music, or some other art. This flattens out after a while, and you land again in your everyday and ordinary lives. From the outside, everything looks like before, but you have an increased inner awareness and ability to observe. Headaches and insomnia can occur in some people when Kundalini wakes up.

It is easy to confuse the awakening of our chakras, nadis, and sushumna with a Kundalini rise. When the chakra is opened, you get experiences that are usually pleasant and satisfying. They are rarely nasty or scary. When you get enjoyable experiences during meditation or the kirtan or can feel the presence of your guru, it is a chakra awakening that takes place, not Kundalini.

When sushumna wakes up, you can experience the spine shining or a streak of light. You can also have sensual experiences that can seem very confusing and illogical. You can smell, hear screams or cry, feel warm, or experience pain. Sometimes, you can get disease symptoms and fever that doctors can not diagnose. When Sushumna wakes up, you go through a form of depression, anorexia, and loneliness. You begin to understand your inner being, your true nature. Materia is experienced as nothing, and the body feels as if it were made of air, or you can feel as if you are not a part of the body. You can communicate with your surroundings, trees, animals, and water. You can start to anticipate things, but usually only boredom, accidents, and disasters. You can feel reluctant to do work, and it is good if, at this stage, you can be close to your guru to explain what is happening.

Fine visions and experiences are not always a sushumna or Kundalini awakening. It can still be chakras that open up or experiences of samskaras and archetypes that emerge due to the sadhana that one follows. But to sum it up, a Kundalini awakening always creates more abilities, siddhis. If you slowly begin to understand the language better, you suddenly start to understand complicated things, become good at cook-

ing, get a hearing in music, etc. A gradual Kundalini awakening is taking place. If you experience temporary sensations and powerful light phenomena or visions, other things may be connected to your chakras.

DIET

When Kundalini is awakened, it is essential to follow a proper diet as the food affects the mind and human nature. During awakening, physical changes occur in the body, mainly in the digestive system. The body's internal temperature drops drastically, much lower than the outer body temperature. Metabolism is slow, and oxygen consumption decreases. The food must, therefore, be easy to break down.

The best is cooked food. Crushed wheat, barley, lentils, and dal are preferred, preferably in liquid form. Fatty and heavy foods should be avoided, and the amount of protein should be kept to a minimum, as they strain the liver and require a lot of energy to break down. When the mind changes, the liver works hard. It is good to increase the carbohydrates in the diet, such as rice, potatoes, wheat, and corn. These cause the internal body temperature to grow and do not require much energy to digest.

Spices play a vital role in a Kundalini yogi. Coriander, cumin, anise, black pepper, green pepper, cayenne, mustard seeds, cardamom, cinnamon, etc. support digestion. They store vital energy and keep the internal body temperature.

KRIYA YOGA

Awakening Kundalini is complex. Most yogic and religious paths are based on many rules that require incredible self-discipline. In the tantric tradition, Rishis developed a series of exercises that would be easy to follow and apply regardless of lifestyle, beliefs, or desires. Kriya yoga is one of the most potent tantric exercises and the path most suitable for the modern man. Kriya yoga aims to open the chakra system, purify the nadis, and awaken the Kundalini Shakti. Through the various kriyas, Kundalini is aroused gradually. It does not rise suddenly, which would be too difficult to handle.

Unlike other religions and yogic paths that often require robust mind control, one should not worry about the mind in Kriya yoga. Even if you can not concentrate or calm your mind, it does not matter – you develop anyway. Rishis in Kriya yoga believe that control of the mind is not necessary.

"KEEP PRACTICING
AND LET THE MIND DO
WHAT IT DOES.
IN TIME,
CONSCIOUSNESS WILL REACH
THE POINT
WHERE THE MIND
NO LONGER DISTURBS."

It is not always the mind's fault that it is anxious or restless. Hormones, indigestion, and a weak energy flow in the nervous system can be the cause. One should never blame the mind when it is disturbed, not even oneself. You are not stupid, wrong, unclean, or horrible, even if you think evil thoughts. Everyone suffers from these, even the most peaceful and devoted. Trying to push back from the mind and ideas and then see them come back again creates a division and, in the worst case, causes mental illness. There is no good or evil mind. They are both the same. The mind is nothing but energy. Anger, passion, gratitude, and joy are all different forms of the same energy. In Kriya yoga, one tries to utilize this energy without trying to silence or dampen it.

In Kriya yoga, one does not try to concentrate or meditate. Mental control is not the purpose. The mind should flow freely and naturally. Kriya yoga is designed for individuals who struggle to sit still and stay focused for a long time. But – everyone should, whether you are tamasic, rajasic, or sattvic, practice Hatha yoga as a preparation. A tamasic person needs Hatha yoga to awaken the mind and body. A rajasic person needs Hatha yoga to balance the vital and mental energies in the body and mind. A sattvic person needs Hatha yoga to make it easier to awaken Kundalini. In other words, Hatha yoga is for everyone and is a preparation for Kriya yoga. You are usually ready for Kriya yoga if you have regularly practiced asanas, pranayamas, mudras, and bandhas for two years.

There are many Kriyas, but twenty are the most important and influential. These twenty are divided into two groups. The first nine are done with open eyes, and the remaining eleven are done with closed eyes.

In the first group of exercises, you mustn't close your eyes even if you feel very relaxed and have an easy time turning your mind inward. You can blink, rest, and take a break, but do not close your eyes.

The first Kriyan is called Vipareeta Karani mudra. It is a method of creating a reverse process in the body. In Hatha Yoga Pradipika and the old tantric texts, you can read about this process:

This nectar originates from the moon. As the sun consumes this nectar, the yogi ages. His body collapses, and dies. Through regular practice, the yogi should try to reverse this process. The nectar flowing from the moon (Bindu) towards the sun (Manipura) should be returned to the higher centers. When the flow of Amrit or nectar can be reversed, the sun will not consume it. The body will instead assimilate it."

When the body has been cleansed with Hatha yoga, pranayamas, and a pure diet, the nectar of the body is assimilated, and one experiences a higher mental state. The mind is still, and you see and hear everything much more straightforward.

It is said that one can influence and control the structure and energy of the body and thus evoke peace, dharana, dhyana, or samadhi. The various exercises in Kriya yoga, such as Vipareeta Karani mudra, Amrit Pan, Khechari mudra, Moola bandha, Maha mudra, and Maha Bheda mudra, regulate the nervous system. The prana in the body is harmonized and balanced. You achieve a state of peace and tranquility without having to fight against the mind. All this is done by creating a flow of unused and natural chemicals in the body. Amrit is one of them, and through Khechari mudra, you can make it flow.

Khechari mudra is a simple but essential technique used in most kriyas. Turning the tongue upwards in the palate towards the nasal passage stimulates specific glands and bandages, resulting in the Amrit starting to flow—one experiences shoonyata, a state of nothingness, being, and awareness of everything. Body temperature drops, and alpha waves begin to prevail. The mind is completely still.

When you have practiced yoga for a while and have reached the point where you have achieved concentration and a complete inner stillness in body, mind, and soul but still feel that there is more to discover, you are ready for Kriya yoga. A calm mind, relaxed body, and proper understanding result from a spiritual life; however, it is not the ultimate goal. The deeper meaning of yoga is to change the experience's cha-

racter, the mind's pattern, and its perception. Man's purpose in practicing yoga has been to expand the mind and release energy. It is tantra and the ultimate goal of Kriya yoga.

THE CHAKRANAS
Colour No. of petals, yantra
action element & bija mantra

Sahasrara chakra – I understand
dark red, 1000 petals. Aum, Shiva

Ajna chakra
White, 2 Petals
Pyramid

Third Eye
I see
Moon Aum

Vishuddhi c.
Purple 16 petals
Cirkel with Space

I talk
Space element
mantra Ham

Anahata chakra.
Blue, 12 petals
Blue davidstar

I love
Air element
mantra Yam

Manipura chakra
Yellow, 10 petals
Red triangle

I do
Fire element
mantra Ram

Swadhisthana c.
Orange, 10 petals
Half moon

I feel
Water element
mantra Vam

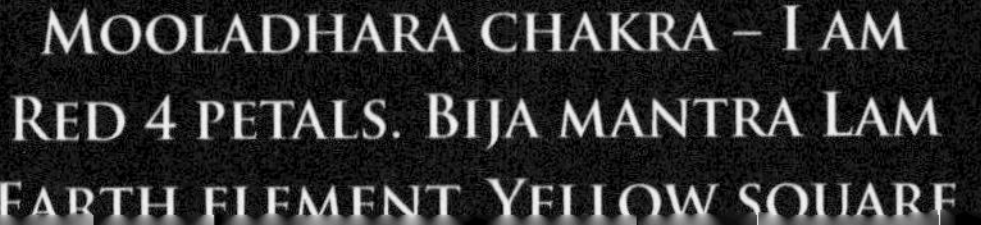

Mooladhara chakra – I am
Red 4 petals. Bija mantra Lam
Earth element. Yellow square

THE CHAKRA SYSTEM

In tantra and yoga, the lotus flower is used as a symbol for chakras. Man's spiritual development consists of three essential phases: ignorance, striving, longing, and enlightenment. In the same way, the lotus flower grows through three phases: clay, water, and air. It grows in mud (ignorance), grows up through the water to the surface (striving and longing), and finally, it comes up from the water and reaches the air and sunlight (enlightenment).

Each chakra is described as a lotus flower with a specific color and several petals. Each chakra consists of six different aspects:

1. Colour
2. Number of petals
3. Yantra (geometric shape)
4. Beeja mantra (sound/vibration)
5. Animal symbol (represents previous stages of evolution)
6. Higher / eternal being (represents the higher consciousness).

OUR CHAKRAS

Our body has many chakras, but the most important ones are along our spine. There are also hidden so-called "Secret chakras."

The eight most important chakras in our body are:

MOOLADHARA CHAKRA

The root chakra is located at the base of the spine and is the chakra that vibrates with the lowest frequency, i.e., the slowest of our seven chakras. Due to its frequency, its color is dark red, and has four petals. The element associated with this chakra is Earth and stands for the most physical and down-to-earth with us.

SWADHISTHANA CHAKRA

The Swadhisthana chakra is about two centimeters above the tailbone and is the center of our sexuality and reproductive ability. It has six petals, orange, and its element is water.

MANIPURA CHAKRA

The Manipura chakra is located at the spine at the solar plexus level. It has ten petals, and the color is yellow. Fire controls Manipura and is associated with will, worldly pursuit, ambition, and career.

ANAHATA CHAKRA

The Anahata chakra is located in the spine behind the heart. It has twelve petals, and the color is blue or green, depending on your yoga tradition. The element air dominates the chakra and controls our emotions and relationships with others. The Anahata chakra is also a symbol of love.

VISHUDDHI CHAKRA

Vishuddhi chakra is located in the neck and has sixteen petals. The color is violet, and the element is space (ether). It controls our communication with the environment on different levels.

AJNA CHAKRA

The Ajna chakra is located in the middle of the head at the pineal gland, and its contact area is the eyebrow center. It controls our paranormal abilities and siddhis. She is also called guru chakra or third eye. It is white and has two petals. It is associated with the mind, reason, intelligence, and intuition.

BINDU VISARGA

According to tantra, Bindu visarga is located on the back of the head, where the Brahmins usually have their tuft of hair. It represents the crescent with a white drop, representing the manifestation of creation, such as consciousness.

SAHASRARA CHAKRA

The chakra is located just above the head and is purple/red. It has a thousand petals and represents pure consciousness. When Kundalini Shakti reaches the Sahasrara chakra, we become enlightened, and according to yoga, we enter nirvikalpa samadhi.

KSHETRAM

The exercises in Kundalini yoga usually focus on the trigger point of the chakra, which has its place at the spine. It can be challenging to experience initially, and many find it easier to focus on the point of contact on the front of the body called the chakra kshetram. When we focus on a kshetram, a sensation is created, passing via the nerve pathways to the chakra and, from there, up to the brain. Mooladhara has no contact point or kshetram.

GRANTHIS

We have three granthis (mental knots) in our physical body that are obstacles to Kundalini. These are called Brahma, Vishnu, and Rudra. They describe the strength of the Maya, the ignorance, and the attraction to material things—the level of consciousness. As an aspirant, one must overcome these obstacles for Kundalini to flow unhindered.

Brahma granthi is in the Mooladhara chakra and is associated with the desire for material things, physical satisfaction, and selfishness. It is also responsible for tamas – negativity, lethargy, and ignorance.

Vishnu granthi has its place in the Anahata chakra and is associated with emotional desires, depending on people and inner mental visions. It is linked to rajas and has tendencies toward passion, ambition, and determination.

Rudra granthi rules over the Ajna chakra. It is associated with the desire for siddhis, mental phenomena, and the image of ourselves as individuals.

THE EVOLUTION THROUGH THE CHAKRANA

Human evolution as individuals and as a race is a journey through our chakras. Mooladhara is the base, and Sahasrara is the very goal or end of evolution.

In animals, Mooladhara is the highest chakra. It is their Sahasrara. Until Mooladhara, evolution takes place by itself and is controlled by nature. When Kundalini reaches Mooladhara, development no longer happens automatically. Man is no longer subordinate to the laws of nature. Man is aware of time and space. Man has an ego; he can think, is aware that he is thinking, and knows that he is aware that he is thinking. Without the ego, there is no double consciousness. Animals do not have a double consciousness. Thus, man has a higher consciousness and must work to develop it. Therefore, it is said that Kundalini lies dormant in Mooladhara until it is awakened for further development.

Awakening Kundalini is a process. It may wake up to return to Mooladhara several times. When it finally reaches the Manipura chakra in a steady state, it will not turn again. What can happen is that it can get stuck in a chakra if there are blockages or if the sushumna is not open. Kundalini can remain in a chakra for several years or even a lifetime.

Before starting to practice Kundalini yoga, finding out which chakra Kundalini is located is essential. The easiest way to do this is to focus on each chakra individually for fifteen minutes over fifteen days. You will notice which chakra is most accessible to experience and stay focused on. Here is Kundalini Shakti.

Awakening our chakras plays a vital role in human evolution. It has nothing to do with mystery or anything occult. When the chakras are awakened, our consciousness and our mind change. This affects our daily lives as our mind controls how we act in different situations, relationships, and emotions.

Today, many children are born with open chakras and Kundalini. When these children grow up, they behave differently. Our modern society often sees these differences as something abnormal, and the result is often mental health care or similar. Going through conflicts within family and work is a common phenomenon. Still, when the mind and consciousness expand, one becomes extremely sensitive to everything in the mind: family, colleagues, and society. You can not overlook something that happens in life. Most people do not see it as usual, but it is a natural consequence of the awakened chakra. Consciousness becomes very receptive when the frequency of the mind changes.

Love, devotion, charity, etc., are all expressions of a mind affected by the chakra in balance. This is why so much emphasis is placed on awakening the Anahata chakra, or the heart chakra. All chakras are, of course, essential to open up, and all have different qualities. Still, you can see that most ancient scriptures emphasized awakening the Anahata, Ajna, and Mooladhara chakra. When Anahata is aroused, we get a deeper relationship with our family and all individuals.

When the chakras are opened, the mind changes automatically. Values change, and love and relationships change character. Disappointments and feelings of frustration are balanced, which leads to a better attitude toward ourselves and life.

PREPARATIONS FOR KRIYA YOGA

Kriya yoga is considered by many to be the most effective method of developing human consciousness. These exercises are said to be those that Shiva gave to his wife, Parvati. Kriyas are relatively simple and must be more potent for the average person to perform.

Before you start practicing Kriya yoga, it is essential that you can feel the chakras in the body, both mentally and physically, and be able to locate its kshetram. One should also know two mental passages in the body, "arohan" and "awarohan."

To develop in Kundalini yoga and preparation for Kriya yoga, it is essential to be well acquainted with the following techniques:

Vipareeta Karani asana
Ujjayi pranayama
Siddhasana / Siddha yoni asana
Unmani mudra
Khechari mudra
Ajapa Japa
Utthanpadasana
Shambhavi mudra
Moola bandha
Nasikagra drishti
Uddiyana bandha
Jalandhara bandha
Bhadrasana
Padmasana
Shanmuki mudra
Varjoli / Sahajoli mudra

IDA AND PINGALA

Yogis have described that man has three leading energy flows in the body. Ida, pingala and sushumna nadi. These can be roughly translated as mind, body, and spirit. Sushumna results from a balanced and harmonious flow between ida and pingala.

Nadis are flows of energy that move throughout our bodies. All the thousands of nadis that flow in the body are connected to the ida and pingala nadi that move along the spine. Every cell in our body, organ, brain, and mind is linked on a mental and physical level, which allows us to speak, think, and act in a balanced and correct way. Ida and pingala nadi are the ones who control the balance between them. By affecting a part of the system, the whole system is affected. This is how asanas, pranayamas, meditation, and the complete yogic system work. Yoga thus affects the entire system of nadis in our body.

Yogis and scientists have come to the same result, albeit with different ways of describing it. Man has two main modes through which he functions. The pattern of the brain is based on ida and pingala nadi, consciousness or knowledge, action or physical energy. Ida and pingala nadis tasks in the three main parts of the nervous system.

A sensory-motor nervous system is where all electrical activity in the body moves within two paths. Into the brain (afferent), ida, and through the brain (efferent), pingala.

The autonomic nervous system is divided into the outward, stress management, energy utilization, Pingala dominant, sympathetic nervous system, and inward, relaxed, energy saving, ida dominant parasympathetic nervous system.

The central nervous system consists of the brain and spine, which controls the two preceding parts of the nervous system.

The yogic techniques are based on the knowledge of our nadis and chakras. The physical experience of these is that you can also experience it physically through the different parts of the nervous system. The nervous system's influence on our physical body describes the importance of balancing and harmonizing the flow between ida, pingala, and sushumna nadi.

THE IMPORTANCE OF PREPARATION, EXERCISE, AND NOT TAKING WATER OVER YOUR HEAD

As a beginner in yoga full of desire and inspiration, it is easy to get water over your head. Yoga is a process in which the body and mind are prepared for more advanced techniques. It's like running. If you have run several marathons, you may need longer stretches to feel the training gives something. You, as a new runner, benefit from running three kilometers. This is precisely how yoga works.

When you have practiced Hatha yoga for a few years, feel comfortable in the positions with all the locks and postures, and master the breathing exercises, you can move on with the most advanced tantric techniques. Then, they will not feel too complicated, and you will have a consciousness that allows you to enjoy the effects of your practice without it becoming too much. If something feels too difficult, go back one step instead. Everything comes to you when you are ready. Hurry slowly.

"YOU EXPERIENCE ALL THE POWER
IN THE COSMOS AND ON EARTH,
IN YOURSELF AND AROUND.
EVERYTHING YOU WANT
IS POSSIBLE
BECAUSE ALL POWER IS YOURS!"

CHAKRANA
INDEX

AJNA CHAKRA

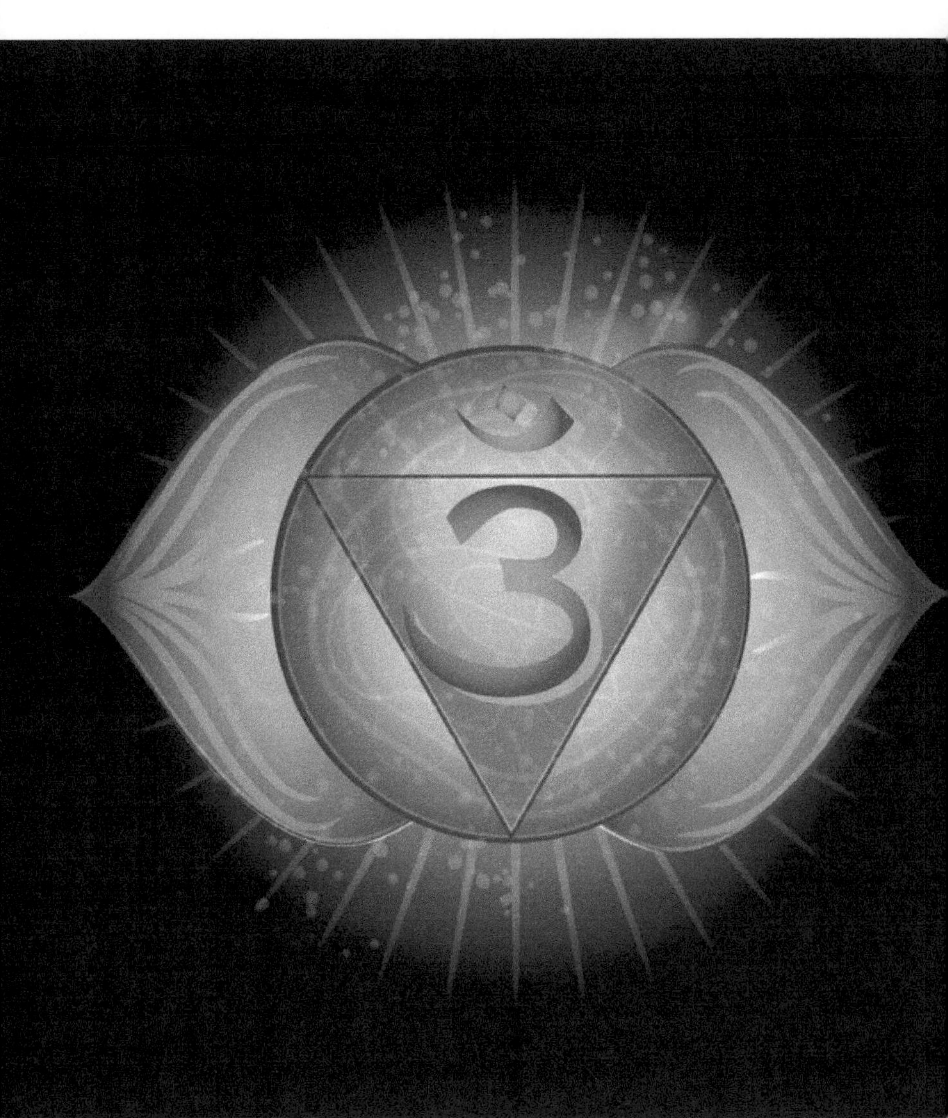

AJNA CHAKRA

TANMATRA *(a sensory experience):* Sense.

JNANENDRIYA *(sense organ):* Sense.

KARMENDRIYA *(body of action):* Sense.

TATTWA *(element):* Sense.

BIJA MANTRA: *Om.*

TATTWA SYMBOL: *Picture of the mantra Om.*

YOGA TYPE: *Jnana, Raja and Mantra yoga (Sattvic).*

LOTUS (PADMA): *White, silver, or smoky with two petals.*

AJNA CHAKRA *(third eye) is associated with the mind, reason, intelligence, and intuition. It is also the center through which two people, through the intellect – on a deeper level, are in contact with each other—for example, the touch between guru (teacher/master) and student/disciple.*

Direct concentration on the Ajna chakra is challenging. Therefore, one focuses on tantra and yoga in the middle of the eyebrow center (the kshetram of the Ajna chakra). This point is called bhrumadhya (bhru- refers to eyebrows, and madhya refers to the center) and lies between the eyebrows where Indian ladies put a red dot, and Pandits and Brahmins put a mark. Various techniques can touch this eyebrow center.

Ajna and Mooladhara chakras are closely related, and awakening in one of these helps to awaken the others. Ideally, Ajna should be awakened to some extent before Mooladhara to prepare the mind for all the hidden memories and impressions that come to the surface as we practice chakra awakening. But the awakening in Mooladhara will also help to awaken Ajna further. The best way to bring about the awakening of Ajna is moola bandha and Ashwini mudra, which are specific to Mooladhara.

The Ajna chakra and the pineal gland are the same, just like the pituitary gland is the physical aspect of Sahasrara. The pituitary gland and the pineal gland are intimately connected, as are the Ajna and Sahasrara. Ajna is the gateway to the Sahasrara chakra. If Ajna is awakened and works, then all experiences in Sahasrara happen as well.

The pineal gland acts as a lock for the pituitary gland. As long as the pineal gland is healthy, the pituitary gland works on a deeper, spiritual level. But for most of us, the pineal gland stops developing when we turn eight, nine, or ten years old, and this is when the pituitary gland begins to function and secrete various hormones that stimulate our sexual consciousness, sensuality, and worldly person. At this time, we started to lose touch with our spiritual heritage. However, through various yogic techniques, such as trataka and Shambhavi mudra, it is possible to restore or maintain the health of the pineal gland. The pineal gland and Ajna chakra have a special significance in esoteric yoga and tantra. It is where siddhis (occult/magical) abilities are manifested.

The" third eye" is a mysterious and esoteric concept referring to Ajna chakra in various spiritual traditions from the East and West. It is also said to be a door that leads into inner worlds and stages of higher consciousness. In tantra and yoga, the" third eye" can symbolize enlightenment or the development of mental images with deeply spiritual or psychological meanings. The" third eye" is often associated with siddhis, such as revelations, prophecy (including the ability to observe chakras and auras), divination, and out-of-body experiences. A person considered to have developed an ability to use his "third eye" is called a Siddha in yoga and is referred to as someone who has acquired siddhis.

HANDS-ON YOGA TECHNIQUES FOR AJNA CHAKRA ACTIVATING AND PURIFICATION

To practice regularly for a month.

Suppose you have difficulty connecting with the chakra's pulsation and can identify with impaired intuition. In that case, there are powerful yogic techniques to cleanse, balance, and activate the chakra. It would be best if you did them regularly for the specified time, and it is recommended that you also follow a healthy, balancing yoga routine to strengthen the effect. Find a form of yoga that you like, and that is at the appropriate level. Avoid caffeine, white sugar, red meat, and stress and energy stealers as much as possible. Also, reduce your internet/mobile usage and give yourself the chance for natural healing. Good luck!

Practice 15-30 minutes.

Shambhavi mudra with Om chanting.
Chakra and kshetram localization/activation and purification through Shambhavi mudra with Om chanting (open eyes – fast Om, then close your eyes and inhale slowly – O … in through bhrumadhya (eyebrow center) … out with M …) Experience the pulsation from the chakra and visualize the color. You can also visualize the yantra.

Anuloma viloma pranayama.

Anuloma viloma pranayama alt. prana shuddhi. Inhale through the left nostril, exhale through the right nostril and count to 1. Inhale through the right nostril and out through the left and count to 1. Inhale through the left nostril and count to 2; exhale through the right and count to 2. Etc. On 5, 10, and 15, etc., you inhale through both and out through both nostrils. If you lose the count, you start again from 1.

Trataka.

Trataka. Light a candle and sit in a meditation position with a straight back. Squint at the light, do not fully close your eyes. Look at the embers in the flame for 30 seconds, then close your eyes and look at the after-image of the flame behind your closed eyes ...

"THE PINEAL GLAND ...
AND THE DMT MOLECULE - THE THIRD EYE ...
THERE MAY BE A WAY FOR THE BRAIN TO TAKE
US TO A HIGHER PLANE OF EXISTENCE, WHERE
WE CAN UNDERSTAND THE WORLD AND OUR
RELATIONSHIPS TO THINGS AND PEOPLE ON A
DEEPER LEVEL AND WHERE WE CAN
ULTIMATELY CREATE A DEEPER MEANING FOR
OURSELVES AND OUR WORLD.
THERE IS A SPIRITUAL PART OF THE BRAIN - IT
IS A PART THAT WE CAN ALL HAVE ACCESS TO
AND IS SOMETHING WE ALL CAN
ACCOMPLISH."

(ANDREW NEWBERG - BRAIN RESEARCHER)

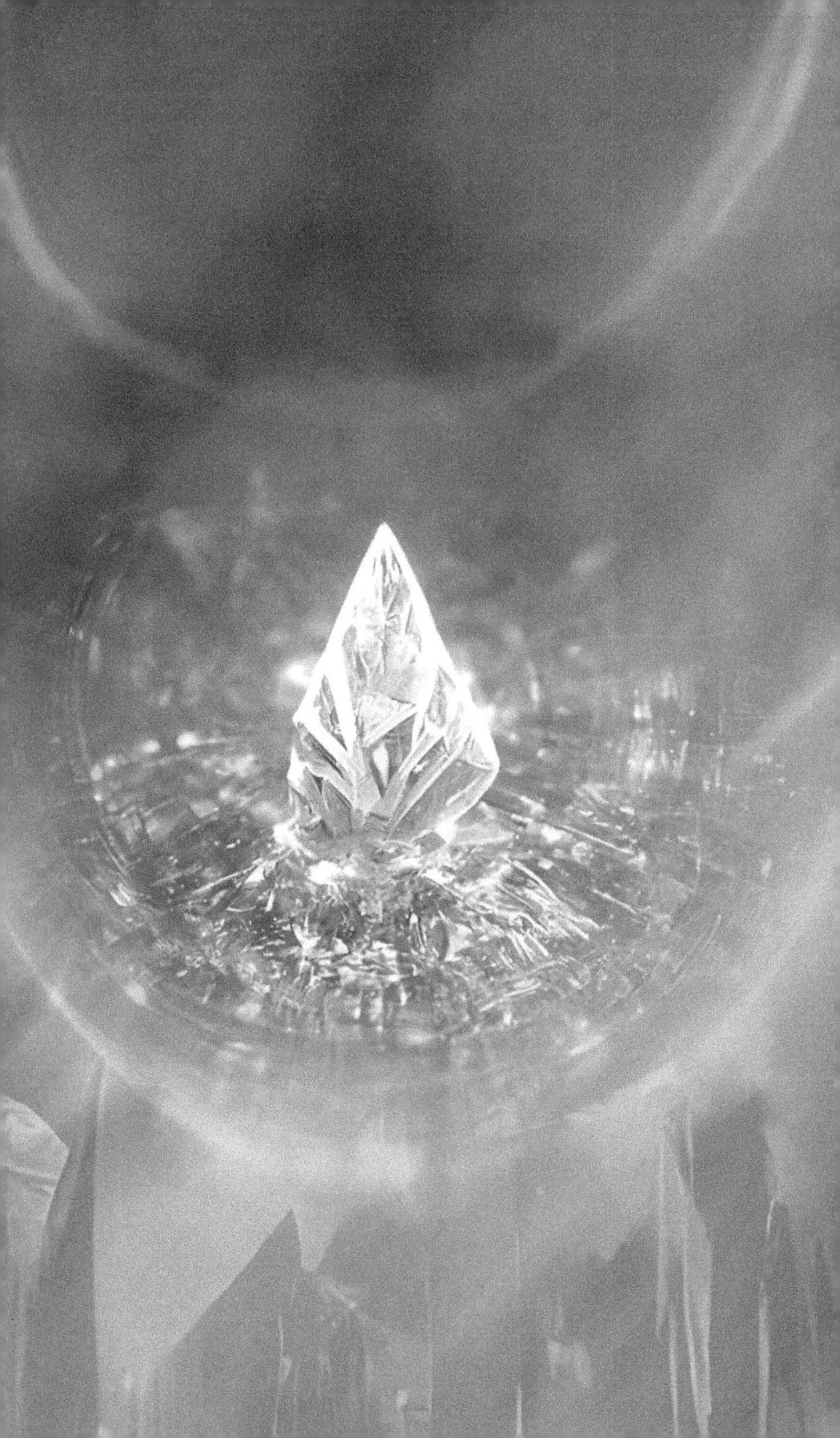

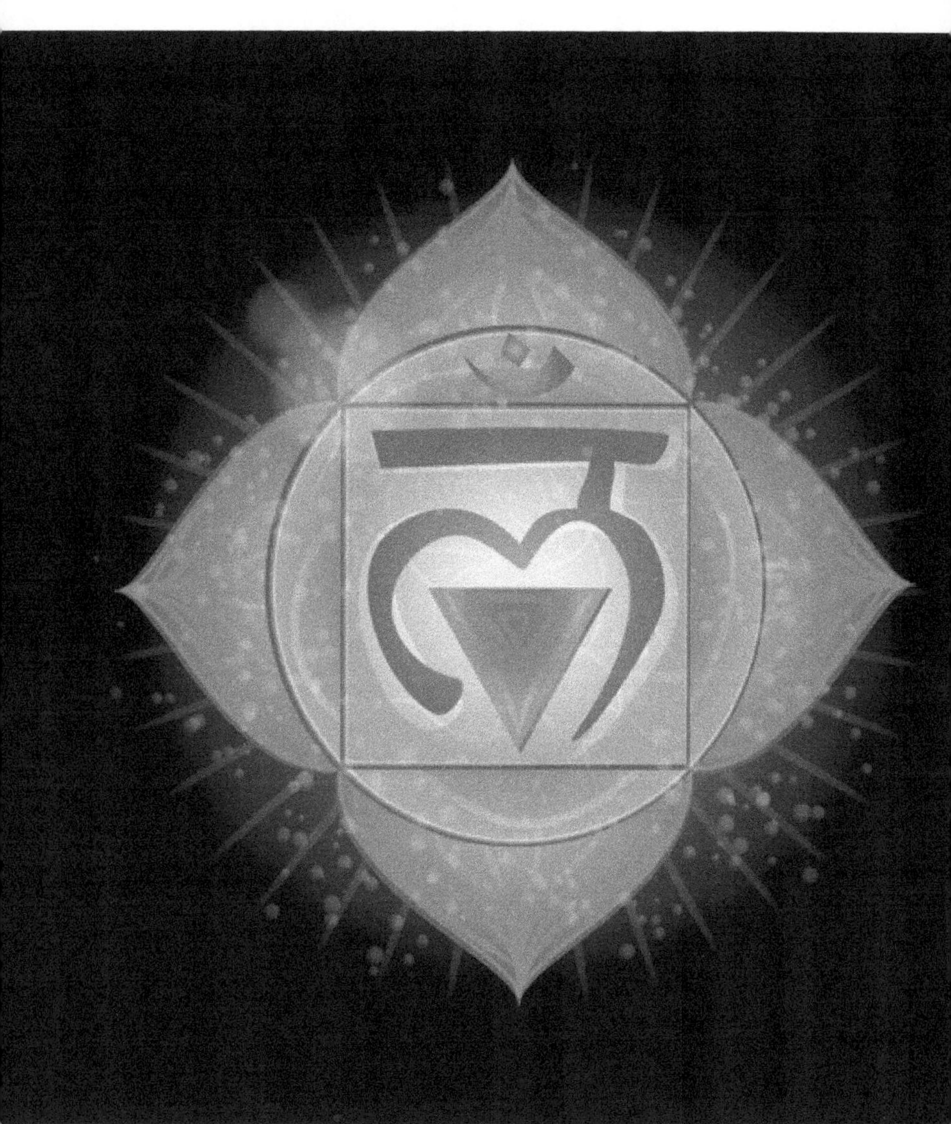

MOOLADHARA CHAKRA

TANMATRA *(a sensory experience): Smell.*

JNANENDRIYA *(sense organ): Nose.*

KARMENDRIYA *(organ of action): Anus.*

TATTWA *(element): Prithvi (earth).*

BIJA MANTRA: *Lam.*

TATTWA SYMBOL: *Yellow square.*

ANIMALS: *Elephant.*

YOGA TYPE: *Tantra and Hatha yoga (counteracts tamas/ inertia).*

LOTUS (PADMA): *Red lotus with four petals.*

MOOLADHARA CHAKRA

Moola means root – a triangular space in the middle of the body at a point between the genitals and anus for men and at the cervix for women. Mooladhara chakra is associated with personal security in both thought and action. At this level, the individual focuses mainly on obtaining food and shelter and securing his reproduction. To create personal security, she surrounds herself with material things, money, family, and friends.

In the middle of Mooladhara, one usually imagines a black swayambhu linga (a symbol of male power, Shiva). Around this, the serpent Kundalini (Shakti, the mother of all prana in the human body) winds three and a half turns – dozing in anticipation of its awakening, as it ascends through sushumna nadi to unite with Shiva in Sahasrara Padma in the moment of enlightenment. This event can only happen when the individual's spiritual development is mature.

MOOLADHARA'S IMPACT ON OUR DIFFERENT BODIES

IN ANNAMAYA KOSHA *(physical body).*
Reproductive organs, perineum, uterine tube.

IN PRANAMAYA KOSHA *(energy body).*
Apana vayu.

IN MANOMAYA KOSHA *(body of thought).*
Security, ownership, safety, survival.

MOOLADHARA IN DIFFERENT STAGES OF GUNAS
Creation and its energy consist of three gunas, fundamen-

tal properties or tendencies: sattva, rajas, and tamas. These three gunas act and react incessantly with each other. The world of phenomena is composed of different combinations of these three gunas. Tamas stands for inertia, rajas for movement, and sattva for balance. When Mooladhara is balanced and sattvic, we are safe and secure in ourselves and the world. When Mooladhara is out of balance and is tamasic, we experience boundless fear. We are in a deep psychosis. As the balance becomes more rajasic, our condition changes, as shown below. The yogi believes he can alleviate and dissolve negative states by identifying one's form with the right degree of imbalance/balance in the various chakras.

TAMAS: *Horror.*

TAMAS / RAJAS: *Anxiety, worries.*

RAJAS / TAMAS: *Greed, self-confidence.*

RAJAS: *Collector.*

RAJAS / SATTVA: *Generosity.*

SATTVA / RAJAS: *Property for good cause.*

SATTVA: *Safe in the physical world.*

ENLIGHTENED: *Unity with the absolute*

HANDS-ON YOGA TECHNIQUES FOR MOOLADHA-RA CHAKRA ACTIVATING AND PURIFICATION

To practice regularly for a month.

Suppose you have difficulty connecting with the chakra's pulsation and can identify with the imbalances described. In that case, there are powerful yogic techniques to cleanse, balance, and activate the chakra. It would be best if you did them regularly for the specified time, and it is recommended that you also follow a healthy, balancing yoga routine to strengthen the effect. Find a form of yoga that you like, and that is at the appropriate level. Avoid caffeine, white sugar, red meat, and stress and energy stealers as much as possible. Also, reduce your internet/mobile usage and give yourself the chance for natural healing. Good luck!

Practice 15-30 minutes.

Moola bandha with bija mantra Lam.
Chakra and kshetram localization/activation and purification by Moola bandha, contraction of the abdomen, first slowly; breathe in – hold the breath … feel the pulsation a few centimeters up from the diaphragm inside the body and pronounce the mantra Lam in time with the pulse beat and then release the lock … then quickly and with Lam in step with breathing. Then, sit for about five minutes with a powerful Moola bandha and feel the pulsation of the chakra

*and chanta Lam in time. You can also visualize the color
and yantra.*

Nasikagra drishti – focus on the tip of the nose.
*Nasikagra drishti – focus on the nose tip without closing
your eyes. If your eyes get tired during this exercise, you can
close them briefly and then return to the exercise.*

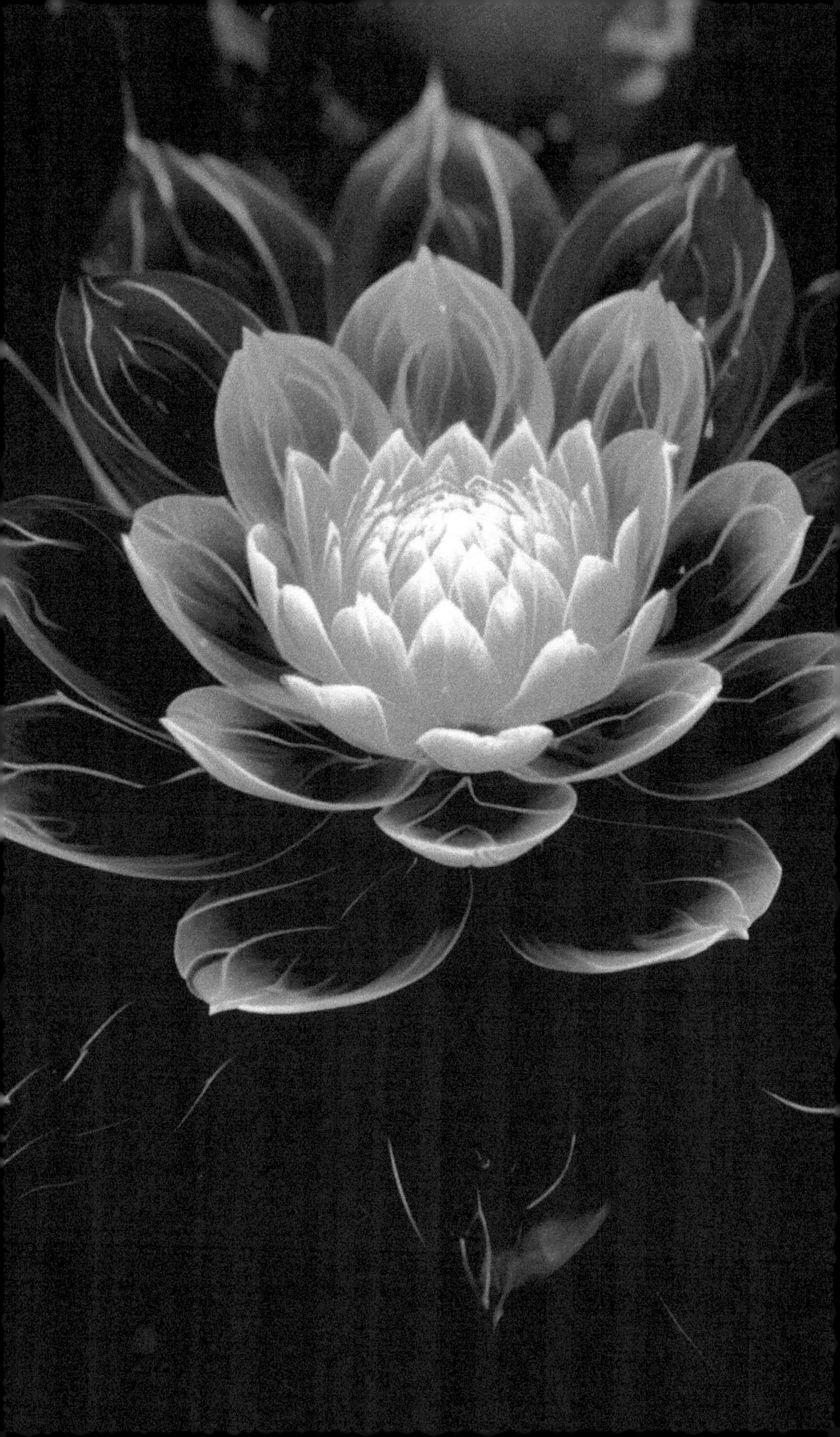

SWADHISTHANA CHAKRA

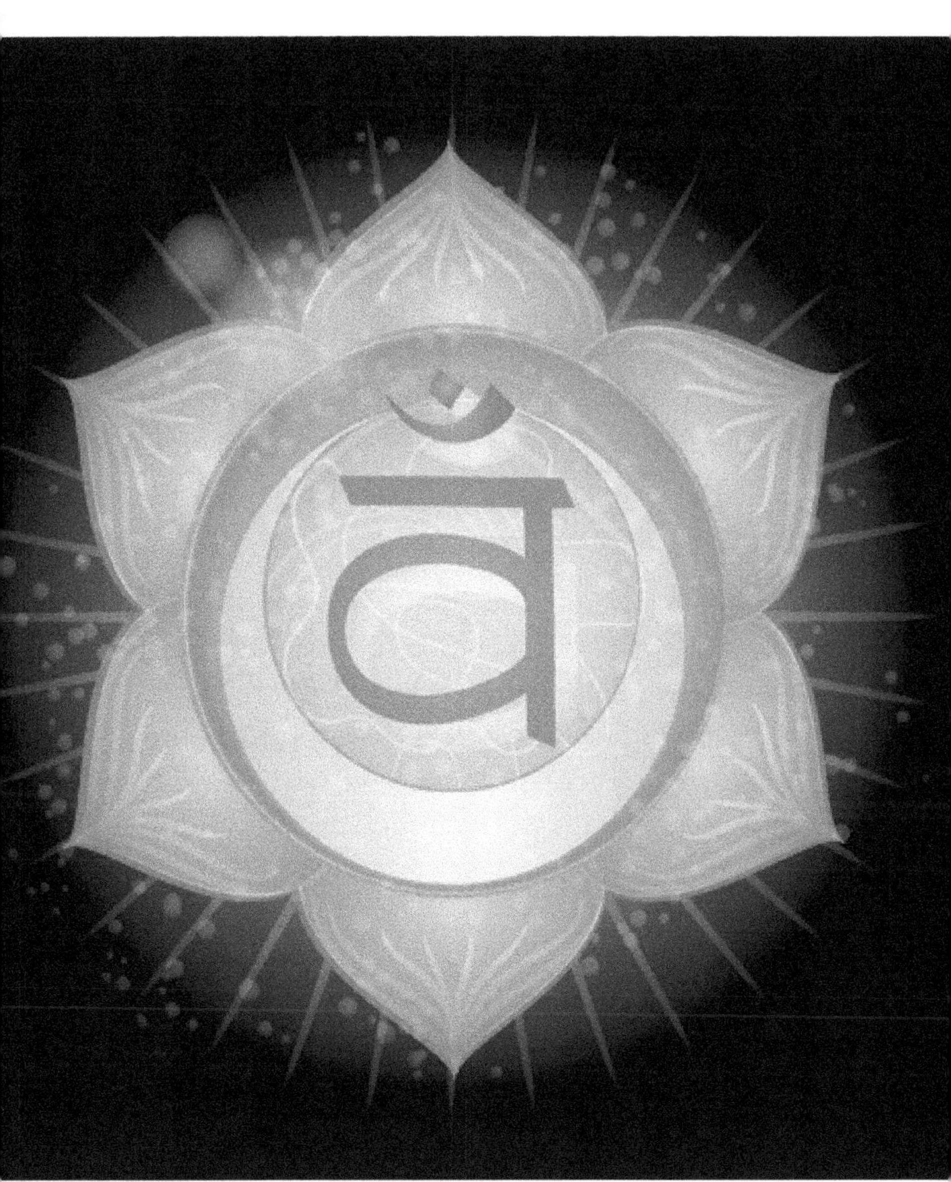

SWADHISTHANA CHAKRA

TANMATRA *(a sensory experience): Taste.*

JNANENDRIYA *(sense organ): Tongue.*

KARMENDRIYA *(organ of action): Genitals.*

TATTWA *(element): Apas (water).*

BIJA MANTRA*: Vam.*

TATTWA SYMBOL*: White crescent.*

ANIMALS*: Crocodile.*

YOGA TYPE*: Tantra and Hatha yoga (counteracts tamas / inertia).*

LOTUS (PADMA*): Orange lotus with six petals.*

SWADHISTHANA CHAKRA *(pleasure, lust)*
The chakra sits at the base of the spine just inside the lower tailbone and at the height of the genitals. Chakra is associated with sensory experiences. One strives to achieve sensory enjoyment through, e.g., food, drinks, sex, etc. You value everything in terms of the enjoyment you can thereby achieve.

The difference from the Mooladhara chakra is that here, we strive for the pleasure of the mind rather than for satisfying basic needs.

It is said that most people in the world primarily act and are motivated at this level. Swadhisthana chakra is also usually associated with the unconscious. It is noted that coexistence – traces or patterns created in the unconscious of our experiences and actions we perform – have their place in this chakra. Samskaras eventually form the basis of the individual's karma. Most of these cohabitants are displaced from consciousness or can even be repressed. Therefore, the Swadhisthana chakra is often associated with desires, urges, and fears over which we have no control.

THE IMPACT OF SWADHISTHANA ON OUR DIFFERENT BODIES

ANNAMAYA KOSHA *(physical body): Genitals, urination.*

PRANAMAYA KOSHA *(energy body): Apana vayu.*

MANOMAYA KOSHA *(body of thought): Satisfaction, pleasure, sex (from happiness to addiction).*

SWADHISTHANA IN DIFFERENT STAGES OF GUNAS

TAMAS: *Depression.*

TAMAS / RAJAS: *Bitterness, the feeling of being rejected.*

RAJAS / TAMAS: *Desire, sexual exploitation.*

RAJAS: *Seeking pleasure, sexual conquests.*

RAJAS / SATTVA: *Humor, caring sexuality with love.*

SATTVA / RAJAS: *Happily satisfied.*

SATTVA: *Bubbly happy.*

ENLIGHTENED: *Ananda, happiness" bliss."*

HANDS-ON YOGA TECHNIQUES FOR SWADHIST-HANA CHAKRA ACTIVATING AND PURIFICATION

To practice regularly for a month.

Suppose you have difficulty connecting with the chakra's pulsation and can identify with the imbalances described. In that case, there are powerful yogic techniques to cleanse, balance, and activate the chakra. It would be best if you did them regularly for the specified time, and it is recommended that you also follow a healthy, balancing yoga routine to strengthen the effect. Find a form of yoga that you like, and that is at the appropriate level. Avoid caffeine, white sugar, red meat, and stress and energy stealers as much as possible. Also, reduce your internet/mobile usage and give yourself the chance for natural healing. Good luck!

Practice 15-30 minutes.

Ashwini mudra with bija mantra Vam.
Chakra and kshetram localization, activation, and purification. For the chakra: Ashwini mudra – first slowly. Inhale, contract the rectum, and hold your breath ... feel the pulsation with Vam in the chakra a few centimeters up from the end of the tailbone ... then quickly and with Vam in time with breathing.

Vajroli (or sahajoli) mudra with bija mantra Vam.

For kshetram: Vajroli (or sahajoli) mudra – first slowly. Inhale and contract the genitals and hold your breath ... feel the pulsation with Vam at the kshetram for the chakra at the genitals ... then quickly and with Vam in time with breathing.

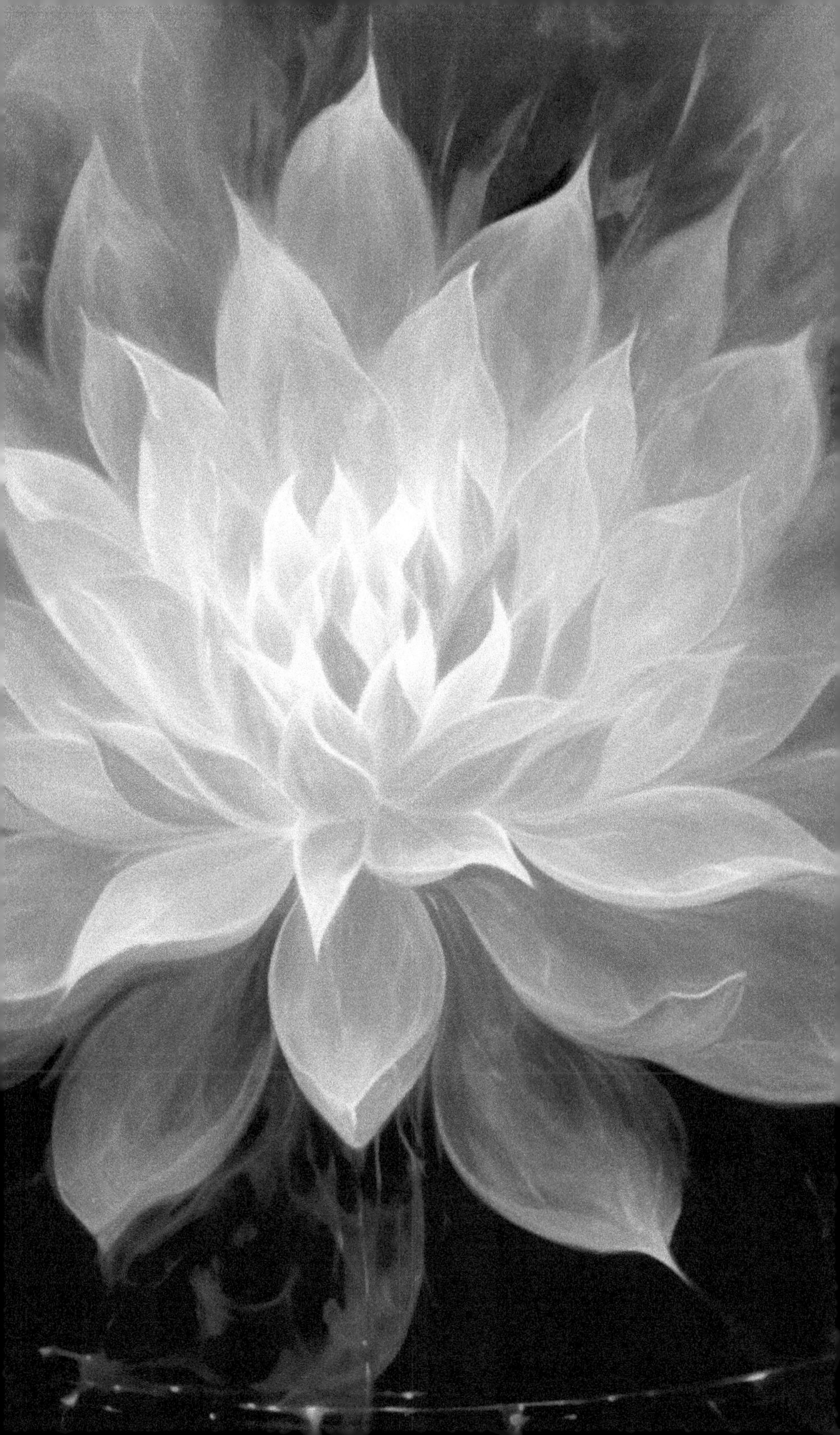

MANIPURA CHAKRA

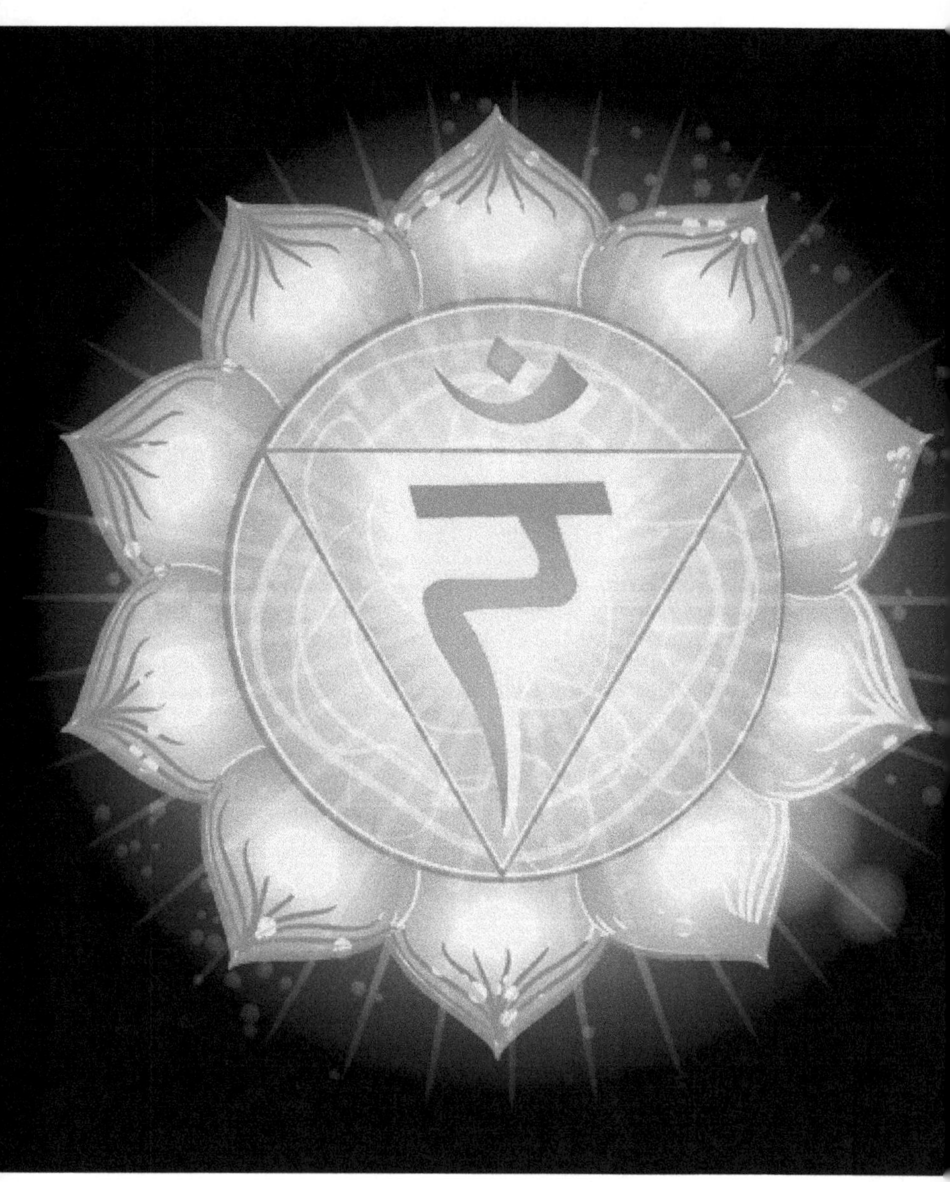

MANIPURA CHAKRA

TANMATRA *(a sensory experience): Vision.*

JNANENDRIYA *(sensory organs): Eyes.*

KARMENDRIYA *(organ of action): Feet.*

TATTWA *(element): Agni (fire).*

BIJA MANTRA: *Ram.*

TATTWA SYMBOL: *Red inverted triangle.*

ANIMALS: *Aries.*

YOGA TYPE: *Karma yoga (counteracts rajas / mobility).*

LOTUS (PADMA): *Yellow lotus with ten petals.*

MANIPURA *(seat of the jewel)*
The chakra is located in the spine at the level of the navel. It is associated with will, worldly pursuit, ambition, and career. Man grows as a social and self-conscious being from the energy of manipulation. She cultivates material desires, such as owning and mastering power, prestige, and usefulness. But also selflessness, social balance, and prosperity.

Manipura's energy is outward and active, a vital energy that provides the power to act and change oneself and one's surroundings. Sometimes, this happens with a selfish attitude where other people are seen as a means to achieve their ambition, but here, the first expressions of a growing self-awareness begin to take shape in man. The ego is still dominant, but the first traces of a genuine, spiritual pursuit are manifested at this level. One begins to question one's existence and one's motives seriously.

THE IMPACT OF MANIPURA ON OUR DIFFERENT BODIES

ANNAMAYA KOSHA *(physical body): Solar Plexus, digestion.*

PRANAMAYA KOSHA *(energy body): Samana vayu.*

MANOMAYA KOSHA *(body of thought): Power, action, self-confidence and striving.*

MANIPURA IN DIFFERENT STAGES OF GUNAS

TAMAS: *Inability to act.*

TAMAS / RAJAS: *Guilt over non-actions, low self-esteem.*

RAJAS / TAMAS: *Frustration over one's inability.*

RAJAS: *Active, brave.*

RAJAS / SATTVA: *Anxious, ready to act.*

SATTVA / RAJAS: *Karma yoga at an intermediate level.*

SATTVA: *Things happen as if by miracle.*

ENLIGHTENED: *Omnipotent.*

HANDS-ON YOGA TECHNIQUES FOR MANIPURA CHAKRA ACTIVATING AND PURIFICATION

To practice regularly for a month.

Suppose you have difficulty connecting with the chakra's pulsation and can identify with the imbalances described. In that case, there are powerful yogic techniques to cleanse, balance, and activate the chakra. It would be best if you did them regularly for the specified time, and it is recommended that you also follow a healthy, balancing yoga routine to strengthen the effect. Find a form of yoga that you like, and that is at the appropriate level. Avoid caffeine, white sugar, red meat, and stress and energy stealers as much as possible. Also, reduce your internet/mobile usage and give yourself the chance for natural healing. Good luck!

Uddiyana bandha with bija mantra Ram.
Chakra and kshetram localization/activation and purification through uddiyana bandha/belly lock with Ram chanting. Inhale, hold your breath as you inhale using the diaphragm, and practice the stomach lock/uddiyana bandha. Experience the pulsation from the chakra and visualize the color while you say Ram quietly to yourself. You can also visualize the yantra.

Bhastrika and kapalbhati with uddiyana bandha.
Inhale and expand your stomach, exhale and contract –

bhastrika; practice this for about 30 rounds, then hold your breath out, lean forward on straight arms with your hands on your knees, and practice stomach locks. The same technique applies to kapalbhati, but now you put all the focus on the exhalation and let the inhalation take care of itself.

Union with prana and apana vayu.
Sit in a meditation position and experience how prana vayu moves down to the navel and unites with apana vayu, which moves up from the anus to the navel on inhalation. Exhale, and the energy currents turn and move up and down the body. Continue for about 5 minutes.

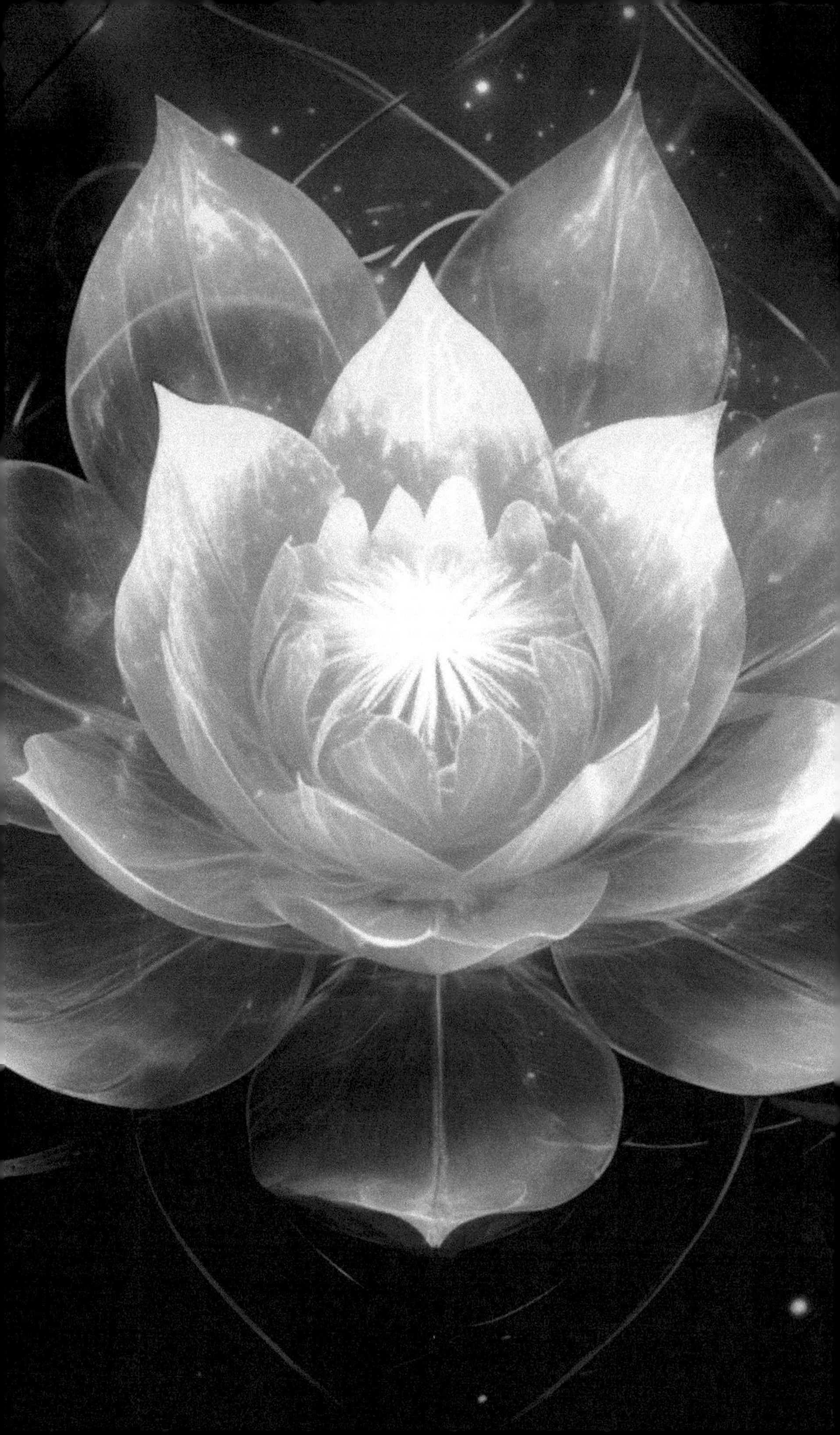

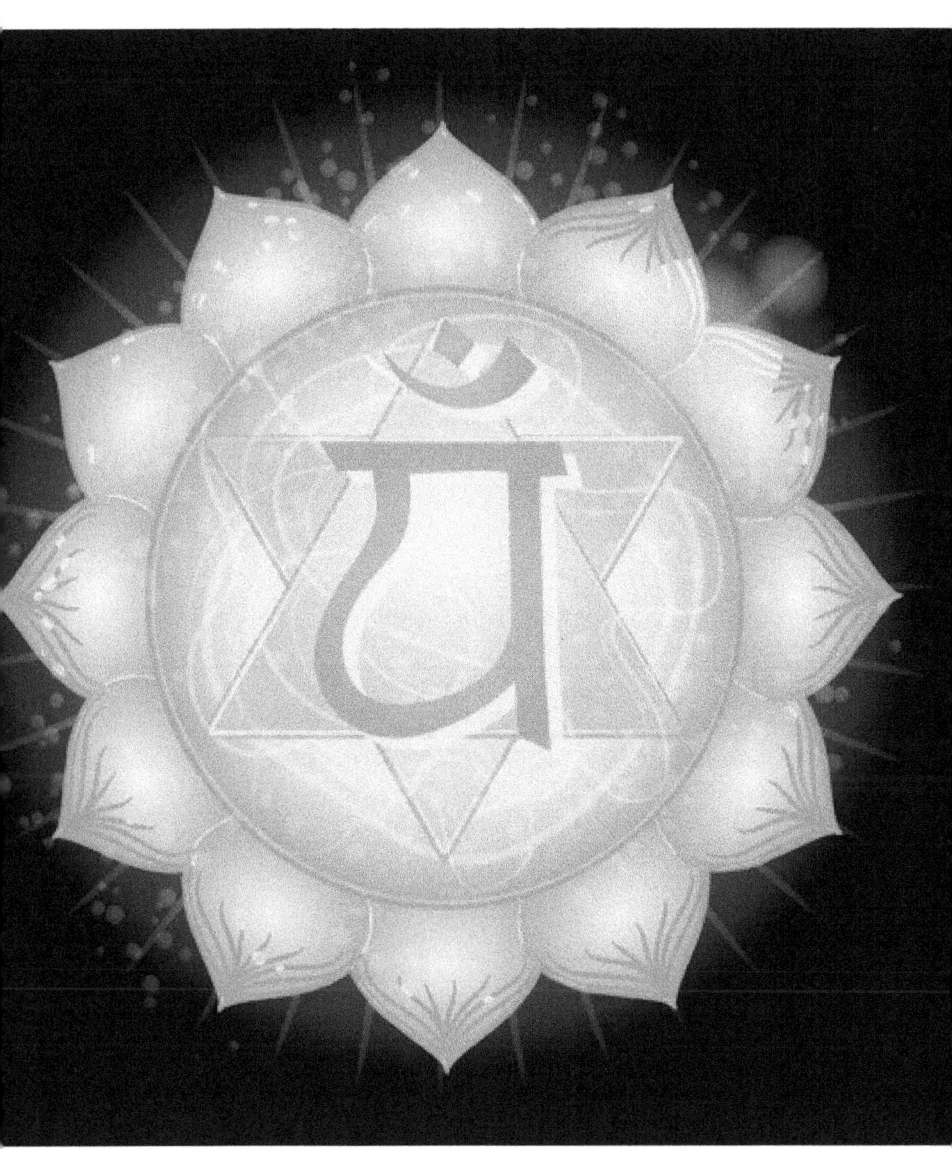

ANAHATA CHAKRA

TANMATRA *(a sensory experience): Feeling.*

JNANENDRIYA *(sense organ): Skin.*

KARMENDRIYA *(body of action): Hands.*

TATTWA *(element): Vayu (air).*

BIJA MANTRA: *Yam.*

TATTWA SYMBOL: *Blue hexagram.*

ANIMALS: *Black antelope.*

YOGA TYPE: *Bhakti and Karma yoga (counteracts rajas / mobility).*

LOTUS (PADMA): *Blue or green lotus with twelve petals.*

ANAHATA *(unspoken" sound," the origin of all mantras). Anahata sits in the spine at the height of the heart. Its energy is associated with love, hate, joy, sorrow, and the beauty experience. Chakra is strongly related to our relationships with others around us.*

At this level, the individual often begins to love everything and everyone unconditionally. You learn to ignore the faults and shortcomings of others and take them for what they are. Anahata also stands for aesthetic discernment and artistic creation. The energy is expressed here in the form of creativity, regardless of which area you are active in. At this level, man leaves the material world to cultivate higher values.

THE INFLUENCE OF ANAHATA IN OUR DIFFERENT BODIES

ANNAMAYA KOSHA *(physical body): Heart, lungs.*

PRANAMAYA KOSHA *(energy body): Vyana vayu.*

MANOMAYA KOSHA *(body of thought): Love, compassion, acceptance and tolerance.*

ANAHATA IN DIFFERENT STAGES OF GUNAS

TAMAS: *Apathy.*

TAMAS / RAJAS: *Fraud, treason.*

RAJAS / TAMAS: *Avoid intimacy.*

RAJAS: *Love under certain conditions.*

RAJAS / SATTVA: *Care about others.*

SATTVA / RAJAS: *Love and compassion.*

SATTVA: *Is love.*

ENLIGHTENED: *Cosmic love.*

HANDS-ON YOGA TECHNIQUES FOR ANAHATA CHAKRA ACTIVATING AND PURIFICATION

To practice regularly for a month.

Suppose you have difficulty connecting with the chakra's pulsation and can identify with the imbalances described. In that case, there are powerful yogic techniques to cleanse, balance, and activate the chakra. It would be best if you did them regularly for the specified time, and it is recommended that you also follow a healthy, balancing yoga routine to strengthen the effect. Find a form of yoga that you like, and that is at the appropriate level. Avoid caffeine, white sugar, red meat, and stress and energy stealers as much as possible. Also, reduce your internet/mobile usage and give yourself the chance for natural healing. Good luck!

Yam chanting.

Chakra and kshetram localization/activation & purification with Yam chanting. Press one finger against the heart and one finger at the corresponding point at the spine. Inhale and hold your breath as you experience the pulsation from the chakra and visualize the color while saying Yam silently to yourself. You can also visualize the yantra. Exhale and then continue in the same way for 5-10 minutes.

Anahata chakra bhedan.

Anahata chakra bhedan i matsyasana. Practice matsyasana

(the fish), inhale through the heart, and pierce the spine and chakras. Feel how the astral body expands like a hot air balloon, and you experience the chakra attributes. You feel light – lighter than air; you float high up in the clouds, experience the blue sky, and experience boundless love and happiness throughout your body, eternal joy in every little cell. When you exhale – you exhale through the spine and heart, and the body contracts slightly. Continue for 2-5 minutes.

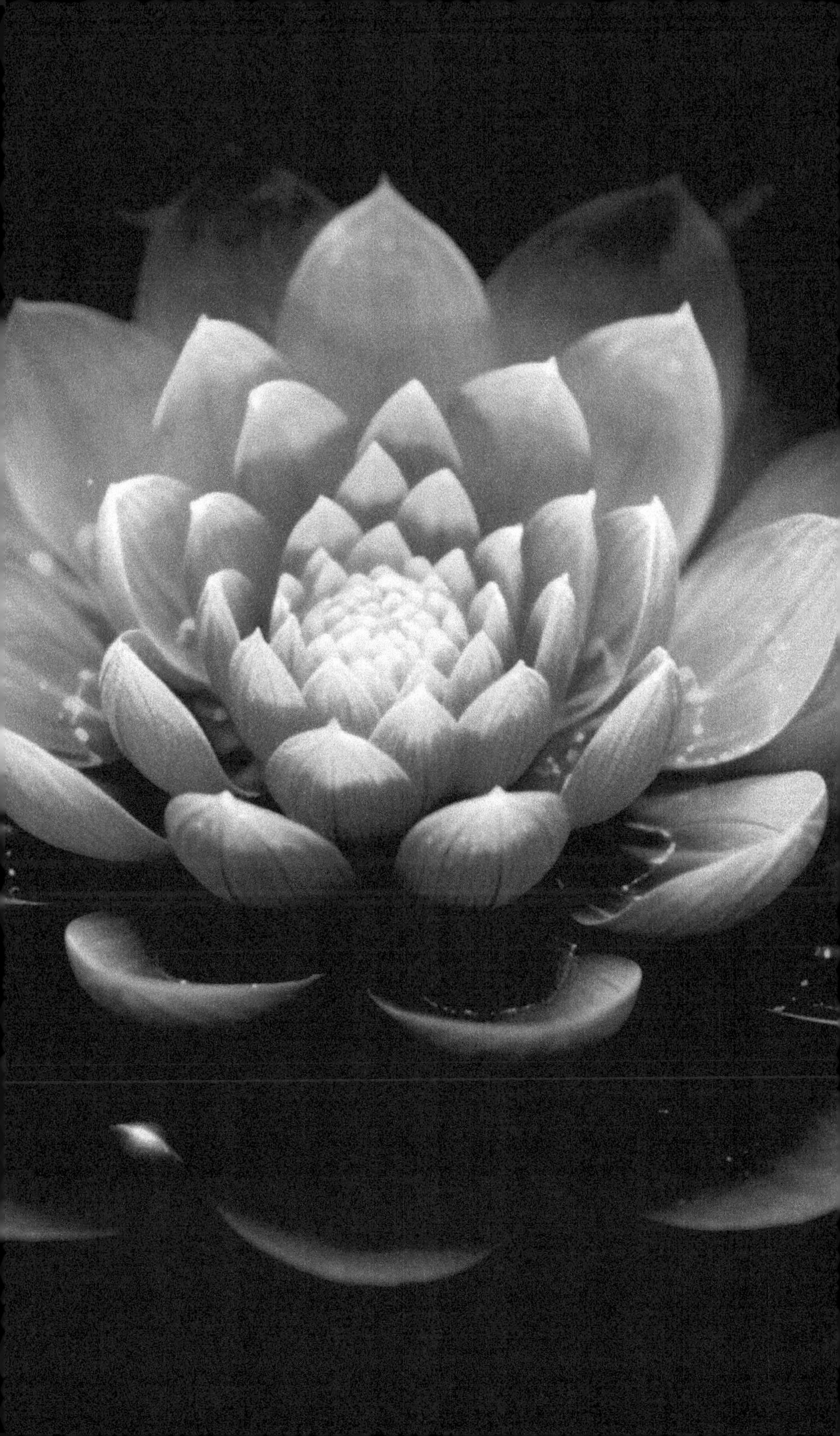

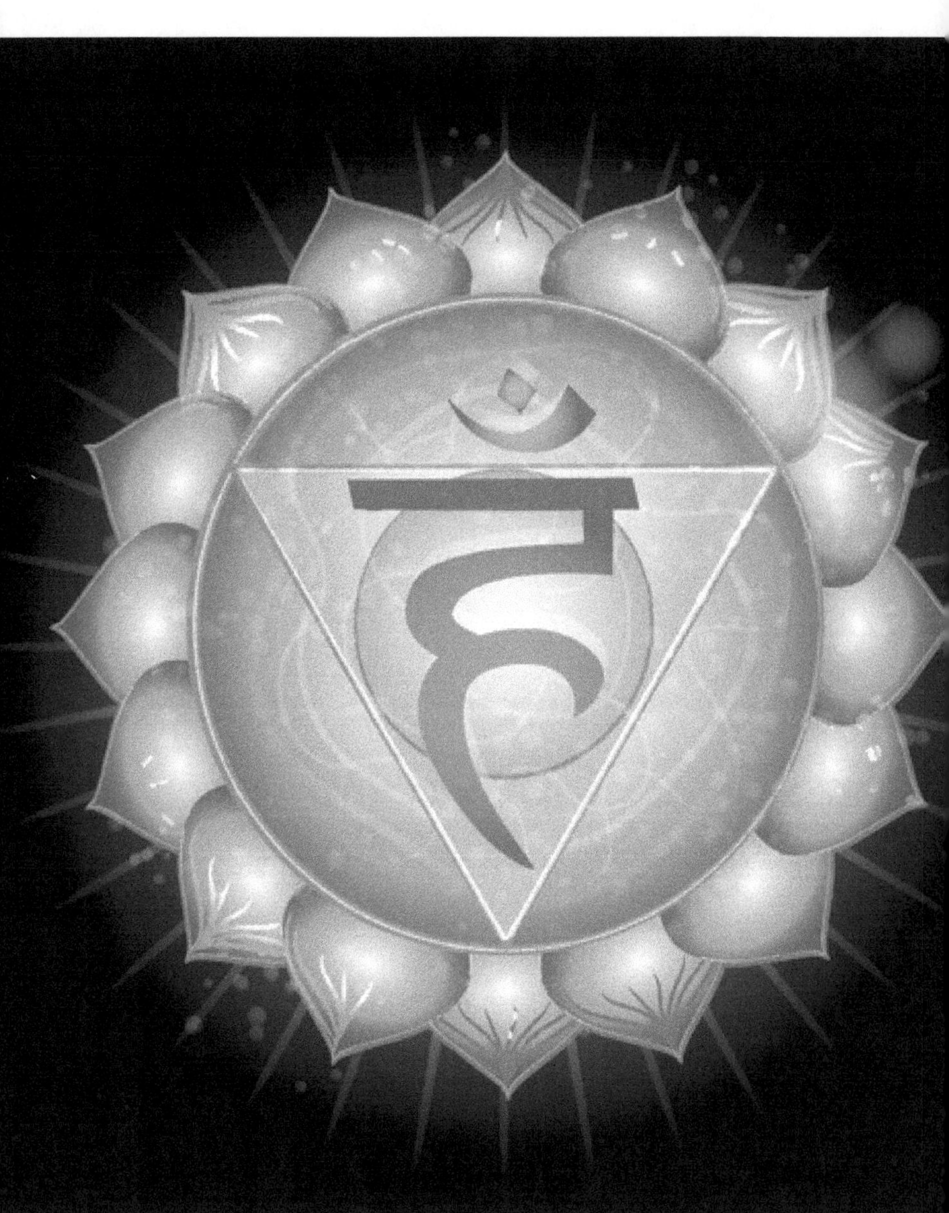

VISHUDDHI CHAKRA

TANMATRA *(a sensory experience)*: Sound.

JNANENDRIYA *(sensory organs)*: Ears.

KARMENDRIYA *(body of action)*: Body of speech.

TATTWA *(element)*: Akasha *(space)*.

BIJA MANTRA: *Ham.*

TATTWA SYMBOL: *White and black circle.*

ANIMALS: *White elephant.*

YOGA TYPE: *Jnana, Raja and Mantra yoga (sattvic)*

LOTUS (PADMA): *Violet lotus with sixteen petals.*

VISHUDDHI *(purity)*.

The chakra sits in the neck behind the larynx. It is associated with an attitude of independence (vairagya), where both pleasant and unpleasant aspects of human life are seen and accepted as rewarding experiences. The world appears as a place full of harmony and perfection. Everything you experience, good or bad, is seen as part of a whole that helps remove personal problems, locks, and limitations and raise consciousness. This attitude leads to discernment (viveka).

Vishuddhi is also associated with expression, communication in general, and the spoken word in particular.

THE IMPACT OF VISHUDDHI ON OUR DIFFERENT BODIES

ANNAMAYA KOSHA *(physical body): The thyroid gland, parathyroid gland, trachea and esophagus.*

PRANAMAYA KOSHA *(energy body): Udana vayu.*

MANOMAYA KOSHA *(body of thought): Communication.*

VISHUDDHI IN DIFFERENT STAGES OF GUNAS

TAMAS: *Isolated.*

TAMAS / RAJAS: *Limited contact / communication.*

RAJAS / TAMAS: *Complaining/whining.*

RAJAS: *Pretty good communicator.*

RAJAS / SATTVA: *Eloquent.*

SATTVA / RAJAS: *Persuader, non-violent communication.*

SATTVA: *True communication.*

ENLIGHTENED: *Cosmic communication.*

HANDS-ON YOGA TECHNIQUES FOR VISHUDDHI CHAKRA ACTIVATING AND PURIFICATION:

To practice regularly for a month.

Suppose you have difficulty connecting with the chakra's pulsation and can identify with the imbalances described. In that case, there are powerful yogic techniques to cleanse, balance, and activate the chakra. It would be best if you did them regularly for the specified time, and it is recommended that you also follow a healthy, balancing yoga routine to strengthen the effect. Find a form of yoga that you like, and that is at the appropriate level. Avoid caffeine, white sugar, red meat, and stress and energy stealers as much as possible. Also, reduce your internet/mobile usage and give yourself the chance for natural healing. Good luck!

Chakra and kshetram localization/activation and purification with Ham chanting.

Press one finger against the neck and one finger at the corresponding point on the other side of the neck. Inhale and hold your breath as you experience the pulsation from the chakra and visualize the color while saying Ham silently to yourself. You can also visualize the yantra. Exhale and then continue in the same way for 5-10 minutes.

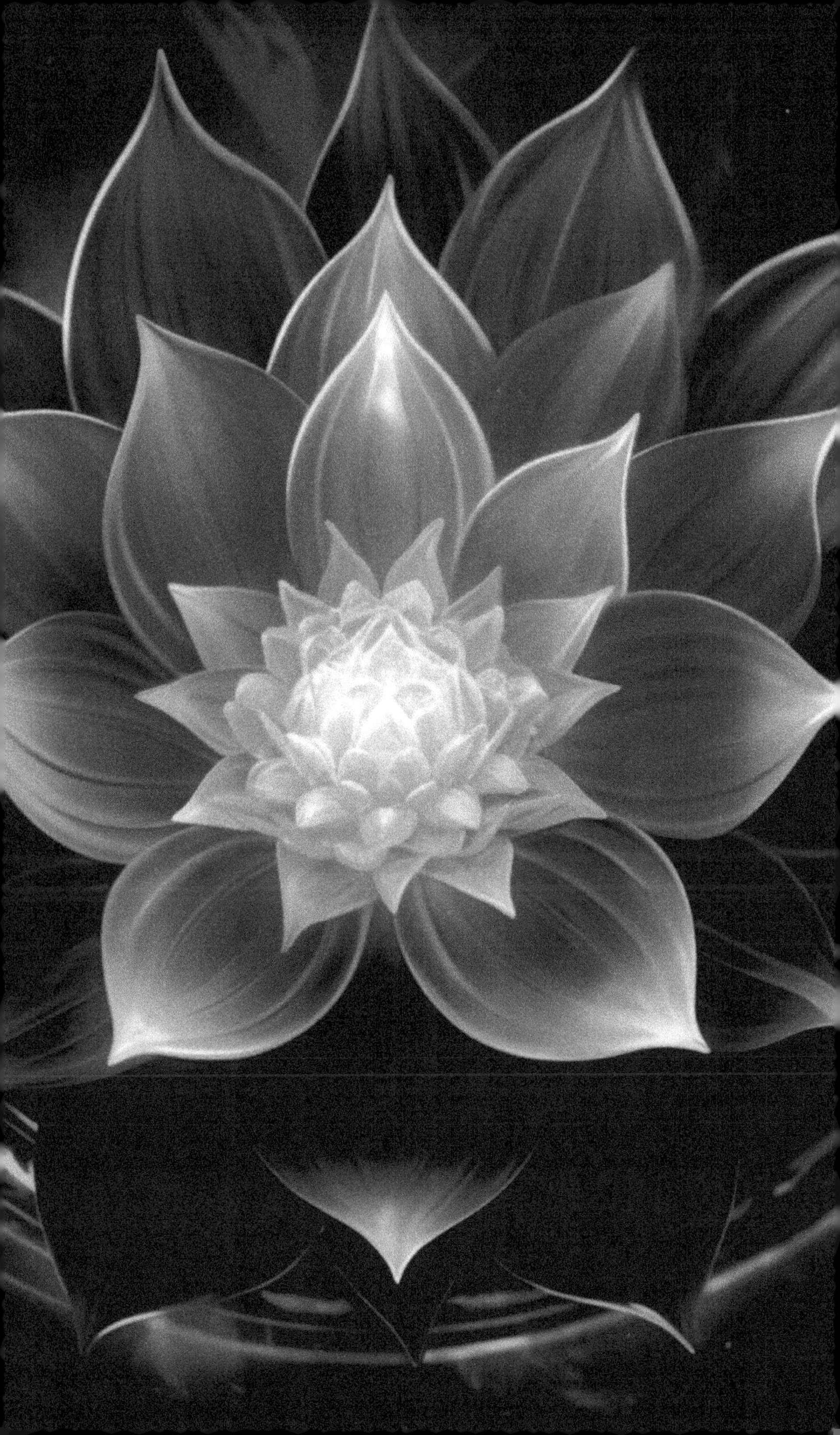

BINDU VISARGA

Bindu visarga is located on top of the back of the head. Many claim that one can not find Bindu in the physical body but can only be experienced via nada, i.e., via its vibration or sound. It is not a chakra in the ordinary sense.

Through techniques like moorcha pranayama and vajroli / sahajoli mudra, we can develop the experience of nada. Through methods like bhramari pranayama and shanmukhi mudra, we can follow nada to its source – Bindu.

There is a close relationship between the Swadhisthana chakra and the Bindu because Bindu is the point where the vibration and sound of the individual creation are first manifested, and Swadhisthana is the center of composition in the form of sexual reproduction. Swadhisthana expresses our physical desire for union with the cosmic consciousness. Sperm and menstruation are physical expressions of the drops of Amrit – the nectar drops of creation or secretions that drip from the Bindu and are burned in the Manipura chakra via the Vishuddhi chakra. The drops control the creation process and the body's aging.

It is commonly believed that Bindu Visarga has no kshetram – contact point.

HANDS-ON YOGA TECHNIQUES FOR BINDU VISARGA ACTIVATING AND PURIFICATION:

To practice regularly for a month.

Suppose you have difficulty connecting with the chakra's pulsation and sound. In that case, there are powerful yogic techniques to cleanse, balance, and activate the chakra. It would be best if you did them regularly for the specified time, and it is recommended that you also follow a healthy, balancing yoga routine to strengthen the effect. Find a form of yoga that you like, and that is at the appropriate level. Avoid caffeine, white sugar, red meat, and stress and energy stealers as much as possible. Also, reduce your internet/mobile usage and give yourself the chance for natural healing. Good luck!

Moorcha pranayama.

Sit in a meditation position. Practice kechari mudra. Inhale – slowly and deeply, through both nostrils with ujjayi pranayama while tilting your head back and performing shambhavi mudra. Experience the Bindu. Keep your arms straight by pressing your hands against your knees. Then, bend your arms while slowly exhaling with ujjayi, pointing your head forward, and closing your eyes. Then relax completely and experience a sensation of lightness and calm in the body—about ten rounds or more.

Vajroli/sahajoli mudra with concentration on Bindu.

Sit in a meditation position. Squeeze the urethra without activating the ashwini mudra or moola bandha. Pinch for 10 seconds, and relax for 10 seconds. Continue like this for about 5 minutes. Every time you pinch, you experience Swadhisthana chakra at the tailbone and say – Swadhisthana 3 times. Then go via sushumna up to Bindu and say – Bindu, 3 times. Then, return to Swadhisthana and relax. Up to 25 rounds. NOTE. In this context, this exercise should be practiced directly after the moorcha pranayama as these activate and locate the Bindu visarga together.

The experience of the inner sound.

Practice the bumblebee first – bhramari pranayama, for a while. 5-10 minutes. Put your index fingers in your ears, close your eyes, and hum quietly. Then, sit in the same sitting position with your index fingers in your ears and be completely silent. Listen for the first best sound in your head. Then, isolate this sound. You use this sound to increase your consciousness. Just experience this sound – nothing else. After a while, you can hear an even more subtle sound in the background – then you concentrate on this sound and gradually use the same technique to penetrate more deeply into the subtle vibrations of the head—10 minutes or more. Shanmukhi mudra.

Sitt i siddhasana/siddha yoni asana.

Sit on a pillow that touches the Mooladhara chakra. Relax. Then, use your fingers to close your ears (thumb), eyes (index finger), nose (middle finger), and mouth (ring & little fingers). Then release the pressure against the nostrils - inhale, close again with your fingers, and hold your breath. Listen to sounds from the Bindu, the middle of the head, or the ears. Then, go from the rough sounds to the fine ones. Keep going for a short time at a sound. 5-10 minutes. Shanmukhi mudra means – to close the 7 openings (to the outer world and start listening to the inner – mind).

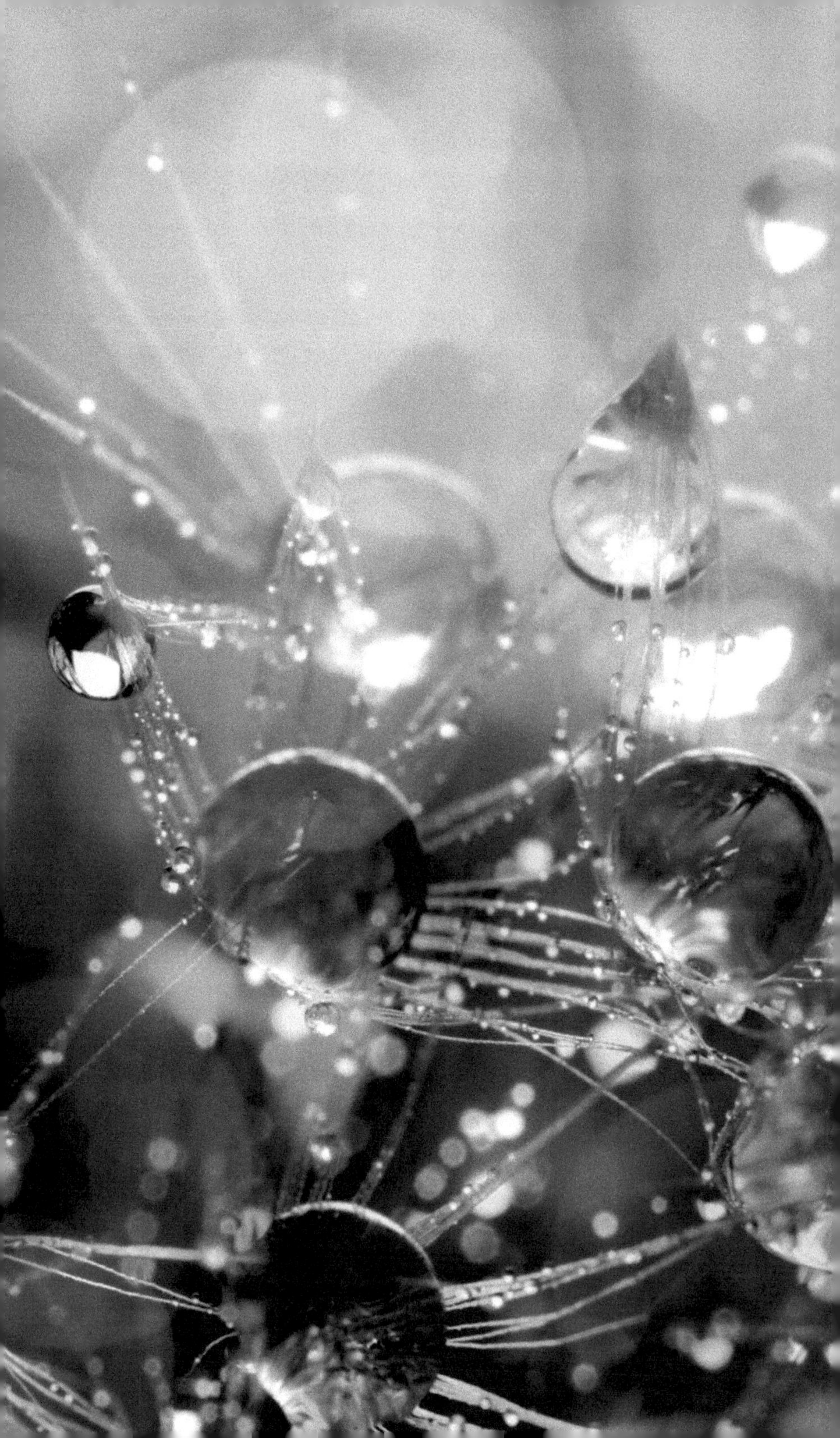

SAHASRARA CHAKRA

The chakra is located just above the head and is purple / red. It has a thousand petals and represents pure consciousness. When Kundalini Shakti reaches the Sahasrara chakra, we become enlightened, and according to yoga, we enter nirvikalpa samadhi.

The function of the Sahasrara is to provide us with other levels of consciousness, which may make us realize that "we are one" and that "everything is one." Through the crown chakra, we experience union with God and the supernatural. The Crown chakra is what is called "pure consciousness."

When one reaches a higher level of consciousness in this chakra, all thinking is released. Here lay the answers to all our questions, the absolute truth that we all dream of getting answers to, and where we find total freedom – We become enlightened.

HANDS-ON YOGA TECHNIQUES FOR SAHASRARA ACTIVATING AND PURIFICATION:

To practice regularly for a month.

Suppose you have difficulty connecting with the chakra's pulsation and experiences of heightened awareness. In that case, there are powerful yogic techniques to cleanse, balance, and activate the chakra. It would be best if you did them regularly for the specified time, and it is recommended that you also follow a healthy, balancing yoga routine to strengthen the effect. Find a form of yoga that you like, and that is at the appropriate level. Avoid caffeine, white sugar, red meat, and stress and energy stealers as much as possible. Also, reduce your internet/mobile usage and give yourself the chance for natural healing. Good luck!

Chakra and kshetram localization/activation and purification with Aum chanting.

Press one finger against the top of the head. Inhale and hold your breath as you experience the pulsation from the chakra and visualize the color while saying Aum silently to yourself. Exhale and then continue in the same way for 5-10 minutes.

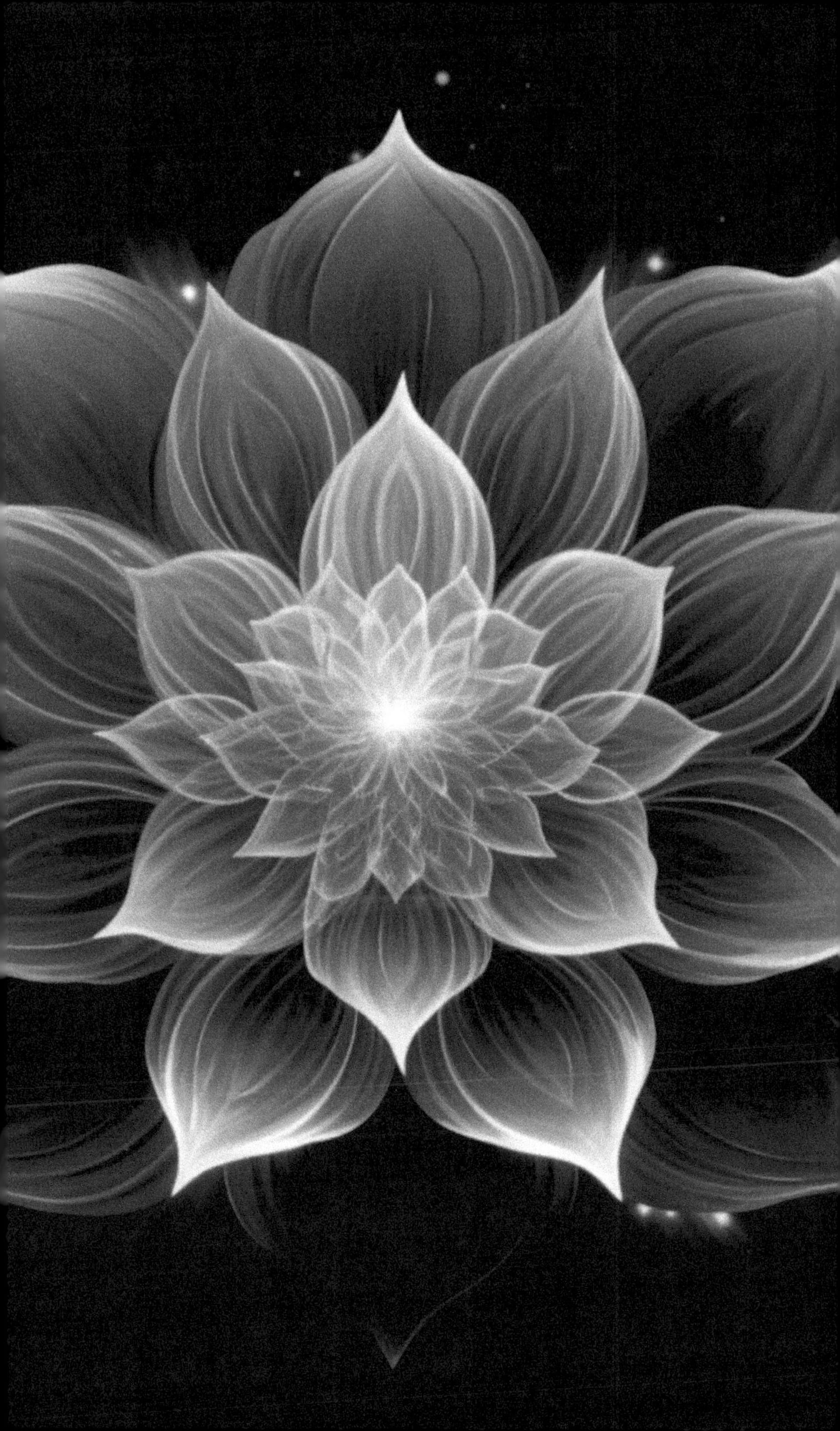

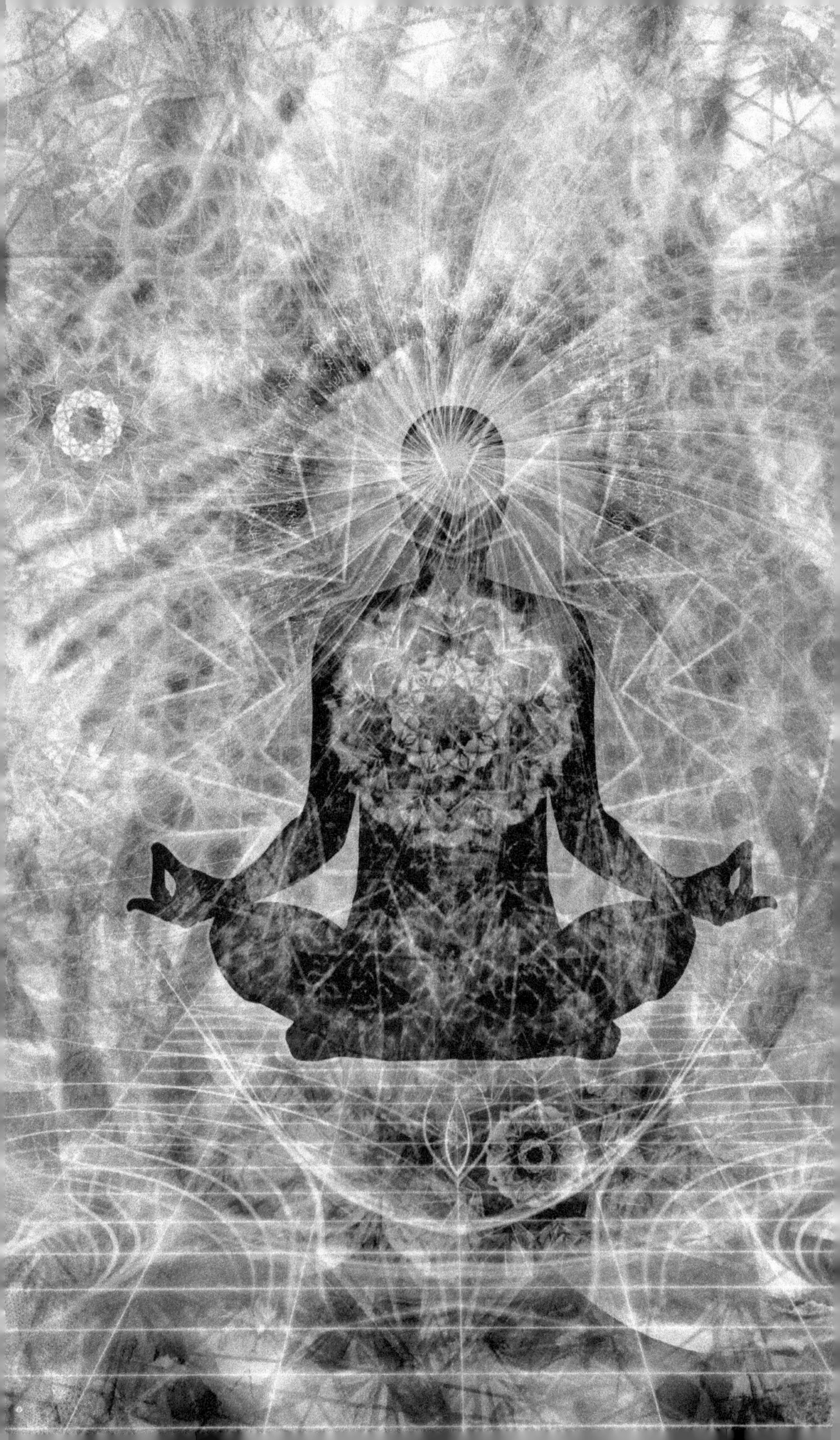

Did you like the book? Feel free to follow me on my social media, share and like, tell your friends about the books, and feel free to write an honest review; one or two lines don't matter. All support is precious. Thanks!

On my Facebook page and Instagram, I post exciting news and tips on temporary offers and benefits you can take advantage of. I often also post my yoga routine and other things related to nutrition and health that may be interesting to take part in. So feel free to join them so you don't miss anything interesting:

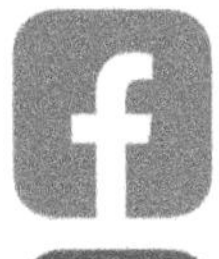 *facebook.com/bhagwanoneofakindbooks*

 *instagram.com/bhagwanoneofakindbooks/*

MY BOOKS AND BOOK SERIES

I have two book series that have different audiences. Great Yoga Books – is a series with the most comprehensive fact books on yoga for those who want to explore the subject in depth. Here, you will also find classic yoga books that are rarely translated, such as Patanjali's Yoga Sutras and Hatha Yoga Pradipika. My second series, Yoga Beyond the Poses: The Ultimate Beginner's Guide to Yoga! covers one yoga topic at a time and is extra easy to read with larger text. For those who find it challenging to read extensive books and want a good and broad overview of the subject quickly. Both series are also available as audiobooks.

★★★★★

TEACHING YOGA
&
MEDITATION
BEYOND
THE POSES

BESTSELLING AUTHOR

Shreyananda Natha

Teaching Yoga and Meditation Beyond the Poses – A unique and practical workbook!

Teaching Yoga and Meditation Beyond the Poses – A unique and practical workbook for aspiring yoga teachers who want to teach yoga and meditation beyond the poses.

Teaching Yoga and Meditation Beyond the Poses is a unique and essential resource for new and experienced teachers and a guide for all yoga students interested in refining their skills and knowledge. Teaching Yoga and Meditation is also ideal as a core textbook in yoga teacher training programs.

The book covers fundamental yoga philosophy and history topics, including a historical presentation of classical yoga literature: Yoga Sutras of Patanjali, Bhagavad Gita, etc. Each of the seven major styles of yoga is described, from Hatha yoga, Raja yoga, Tantra yoga, Bhakti yoga, and Kundalini yoga, to knowledge about the chakras, Ayurveda and magic mantras and yantras. The book provides extensive support and tools for teaching integrated and classical yoga (asanas), breathing techniques (pranayama), deep relaxation (Yoga Nidra), and meditation (Ajapa Japa). The book is divided into eight modules with associated knowledge tests and complete yoga and meditation classes.

https://rb.gy/9s6edj

Download the ***AUDIOBOOK*** *here!*

SCAN QR-CODE or go to:

https://bit.ly/3G8KlsA

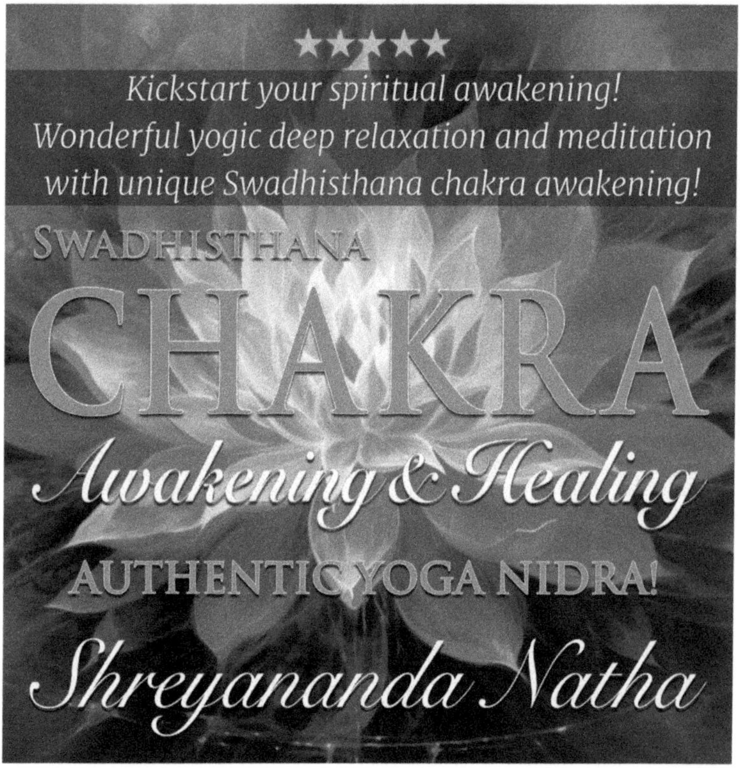

www.ingramcontent.com/pod-product-compliance
Lightning Source LLC
LaVergne TN
LVHW051054180726
843512LV00019B/1468